FITNESS

FOR HEALTH AND SPORTS

FITNESS
FOR HEALTH AND SPORTS

Patricia G. Avila, M.D.

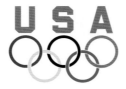

Penmarin Books
Granite Bay, California

Bookmark Publishers
Jamul, California

Editor in chief: Hal Lockwood
Sponsoring editor: Vernon Avila
Production: Connie Hathaway
Design: Mary Beth Salmon
Layout and composition: Trina Stahl
Publicity: Robin Lockwood Public Relations
Printing and binding: Palace Press International
Cover Photographs: All photos © Allsport Photography USA:
Counterclockwise from upper left: Sharon Hanson-Lowery by Tony Duffy;
Tom Dolan by Al Bello; Valerie Brisco by Mike Powell; Kip Simons by D.
Reinzinger; Tommy Moc by Agence Vandystadt; Tara Lipinski by Clive
Brunskill

Editorial Offices: **Sales and Customer Service Offices:**
Penmarin Books   Access Publishers Network
2011 Ashridge Way   6893 Sullivan Road
Granite Bay, CA 95746   Grawn, MI 49637
                                  (800) 345-0096

Penmarin Books are available at special discounts for bulk purchases for
premiums, sales promotions, or education. For details, contact the Publisher.
On your letterhead, include information concerning the intended use of the
books and how many you wish to purchase.

Visit our Website at **www.penmarin.com** for more information about this
and other exciting titles.

Printed in China
1 2 3 4 5 6 7 8 9 10   03 02 01 00 99

Library of Congress Cataloging-in-Publication Data

Avila, Patricia G.
       Fitness for health and sports / Patricia G. Avila.
              p.   cm.
       Includes bibliographical references and index.
       ISBN 1-883955-09-2
       1. Physical fitness. 2. Exercise. 3. Health. 4. Sports—
Physiological aspects. 5. Sports medicine. I. Title.
       RA781.A93   1999
       613.7´1—dc21   99-10291

The use of Olympic-related marks and terminology is authorized by the
U.S. Olympic Committee pursuant to the Olympic Amateur Sports Act
(formerly 36 USC 380, now 36 USC 220506).

Disclaimer: This book is not intended to substitute for medical consultation or the recommendation of your physician. Before beginning any nutrition, exercise, or sport program, obtain medical clearance from your physician, especially if you have any special medical needs and/or are over 40 years of age. Since the field of health, fitness, and sports is continually changing, you should consult with your physician, nutritionist, sports trainer, or other health professional regarding the most recent information on these topics.

To my children,

PATRICK and RAQUEL,

for their love and support

and

In loving memory,

to my father,

ROBERT EARL FRYE,

for his gifts of love, wisdom,

and the joy of fitness

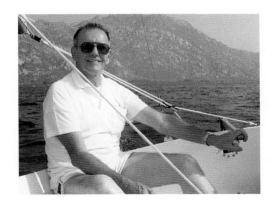

CONTENTS

Part I

THE JOY OF PHYSICAL FITNESS

Beauty 2

Flexibility. 4

Strength 6

Endurance. 8

Longevity 10

Camaraderie 12

Victory!. 14

Part II

GETTING READY

Optimal health 18

    Playing it safe. 18

    The four components of fitness 19

Setting goals 20

    Goals 20

    What is moderately intense activity? 20

    Overcoming hurdles 21

Fitness assessment 22

    Target heart rate. 23

Monitor your heart rate. 24

    Radial pulse 24

    Carotid pulse 24

    Exercise within your Target Heart Rate Zone 24

    Tips for making progress. 25

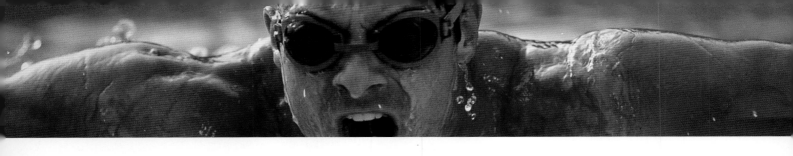

Aerobic fitness 26

    What kind of exercise makes sense? 27

Aerobic benefits 28

The FIT program 30

    Guidelines for aerobic training 31

Muscular fitness 32

Muscular strength 34

    Muscle contraction 34

    Forget the notion "No pain, no gain"! 34

    How to build muscular strength 35

    Guidelines for safe strength training 35

Muscular endurance 36

    Endurance and nutrition 36

Body shaping 37

    Weight control and energy balance 37

    Calculating your energy balance 37

Body composition 38

    Waist-to-hip ratio 38

    Determining healthy weight 39

The food pyramid 40

    What nutrients does each food group provide? 41

Food choices 42

    Eating sensibly 42

    Summary 43

A healthy mind and body 44

    The mind 44

    Breathing 44

    A tip for relaxation 44

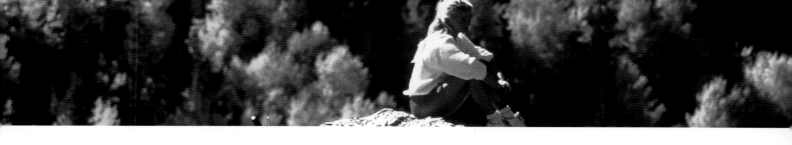

Part III

STRETCHING AND STRENGTHENING

Stretching 48
    Stretching for flexibility 48
    How to stretch. 49
    Overall body stretch. 49
Upper body 50
    Neck stretches 50
    Shoulder and upper back stretches 50
    Chest and upper back stretch 51
    Triceps and shoulder stretch 51
    Profile: Sally Scovel, Rowing 51
Back and hips. 52
    Lower back stretch. 52
    Hip and back stretch 53
    Profile: Karen Dunne, Cycling 53
Upper legs 54
    Hamstring stretch 54
    Profile: Tim Seaman, Race Walking 54
    Quadriceps stretches 55
    Hip and groin stretch 55
Lower legs and feet. 56
    Standing calf stretch. 56
    Calf and Achilles tendon stretch 56
    Sitting calf stretch 56
    Ankle and foot stretch 57
    Foot arch stretch 57
    Profile: Kevin Fitzpatrick, Discus 57

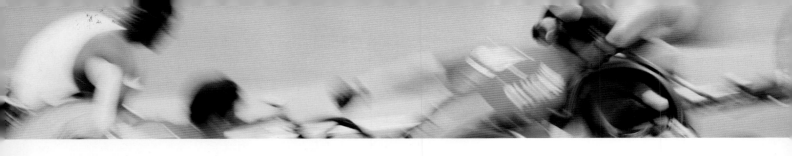

Strengthening 58
    Strengthening exercises. 58
    Strengthening program. 59
    Dangers of anabolic steroids. 59
Back and shoulders. 60
    Strengthening the back and shoulders 60
    Profile: Michelle Borkhuis, Rowing. 60
    Strengthening the arms and chest 61
Arms 62
    Strengthening the biceps. 62
    Strengthening the biceps and forearms 62
    Strengthening the triceps 63
    Strengthening the fingers, hands, wrists, and forearms 63
    Profile: Jo-Ann Malahy, Archery. 63
Abdominals 64
    Strengthening the abdominal muscles 64
    Profile: Pete Kelly, Weight Lifting. 65
Hips and legs 66
    Strengthening the hip extensor and gluteals. 66
    Strengthening the quadriceps 66
    Strengthening the hip abductor and outer thigh. 67
    Profile: Steve Danielson, Field Hockey 67
Legs 68
    Strengthening the inner thigh 68
    Strengthening the lower leg 68
Combinations. 69
    Strengthening the arms and legs and improving coordination. 69

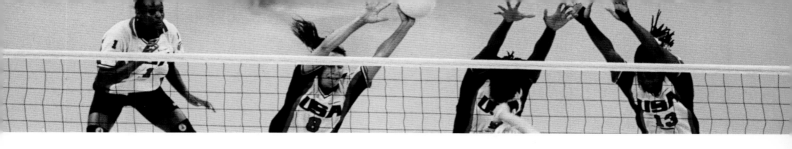

Part IV

SPORTS INJURIES

Understanding injury 72
  Defining a sports injury 73
  Rating injury severity 74
    CHART: INJURY SEVERITY GUIDELINES 75
    Caring for injuries 76
    What you can do for a mild to moderate injury 76
    Over-the-counter medication 76
    Prevention 77
  Soft tissue injuries 78
    The human muscular system 78
    CHART: COMMON SOFT TISSUE INJURIES 80
  Skeletal injuries 82
    Fractures 82
    CHART: GENERAL HEALING TIMES FOR SPRAINS AND FRACTURES . . 82
    Dislocations 83
    Stress fractures 83
  Other sport-related injuries 84
Prevention, care, and rehabilitation 86
  Head and neck 88
    Anatomy of the head and neck 88
    Preventing head and neck injuries 89
    Common head and neck injuries 90
    Profile: Courtney DeBolt, Volleyball 93
  Shoulders, upper back, and chest 94
    Anatomy of the shoulders, upper back, and chest 94
    Preventing shoulder injuries 96
    Common shoulder injuries 97
    Profile: Sabir Muhammad, Swimming 99

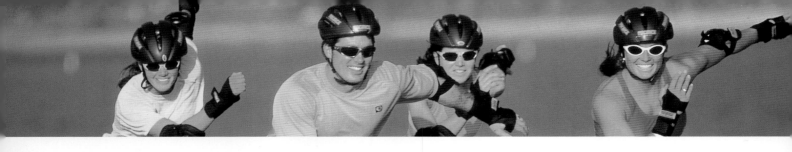

Upper extremities. 100
   Anatomy of the upper extremities 100
   Preventing upper extremity injuries 101
   Common upper extremity injuries 102
   Profile: Emily Dirksen, Rowing 105
Abdomen. 106
   Anatomy of the abdomen 106
   Preventing abdominal injuries 107
   Common abdominal injuries 107
   Profile: Al Oerter, Discus. 108
Lower back and hips 109
   Anatomy of the lower back and hips 109
   Preventing lower back and hip injuries. 110
   Common injuries of the lower back and hips 110
   Profile: Tyrone Scott, Triple Jump 113
Thigh 114
   Anatomy of the thigh 114
   Preventing thigh injuries 115
   Common thigh injuries 116
   Profile: Blaine Wilson, Gymnastics. 118
Knee 119
   Anatomy of the knee. 119
   Preventing knee injuries. 120
   Common knee injuries. 122
   Profile: Picabo Street, Skiing 124
Lower leg, ankle, and foot 126
   Anatomy of the lower leg, ankle, and foot 126
   Preventing injuries to the lower leg, ankle, and foot 127
   Common injuries of the lower leg, ankle, and foot 128
   Profile: Tommy Moe, Skiing. 134

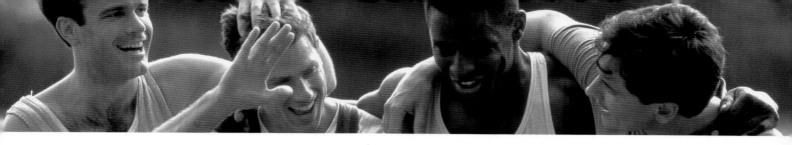

Appendix A
Personal Fitness Plan 135
    Personal Fitness Program Log 136
    Stretching Log 139
    Muscular Fitness Log 140
    Body Shaping Log 141

Appendix B
Body Weight Tables 142
    Body Mass Index 142
    Metropolitan Life Insurance Company Tables 144
        Desirable Weights for Men and Women 144
        Average Values for Body Fat According to Age and Gender 144
        Recommended Calorie Consumption for Adult Males 145
        Recommended Calorie Consumption for Adult Females 146

Appendix C
Nutrition and Weight Control 147
    Five positive steps to successful weight control 147
    Healthy eating: A daily food guide 147
    Serving size 148
    Sample menus 149
    Daily U.S. recommended dietary allowances
        (RDA) for vitamins and minerals 151

Appendix D
Hydration and Heat Stress 153
    Hydration 153
    Heat stress 153

Appendix E
Protecting Your Skin from the Sun. 155
   Preventive measures 155
   Self-examination. 155

Appendix F
Workout Apparel and Athletic Shoes 157
   Winter workout clothes. 157
   Summer workout clothes. 157
   Buying athletic shoes. 157

Appendix G
Relaxation Techniques 159
   Breathing 159
   Visualization. 159
   Belly breathing 159

Appendix H
Preventive Medicine Guidelines. 160

Appendix I
Preventing Infections Transmitted by Blood 162

Resources 163
Bibliography and Websites. 169
About the U.S. Olympic Committee 173
The Sports Medicine Division 177
Index 181

ABOUT THE AUTHOR

Patricia G. Avila, M.D., M.P.H., is one of the primary care and preventive medicine physicians for the USOC's ARCO Olympic Training Center in Chula Vista, California. She also has an active private practice in preventive and family medicine in Coronado, California.

Before her medical training, Dr. Avila taught human anatomy, physiology, and physiological psychology in the San Diego Community Colleges. She received her M.D. degree from UCC, Cayey, Puerto Rico, interned at Georgetown University in internal medicine, and completed her residency at UC San Diego / San Diego State University in general preventive medicine. She is currently part of the Sharp family practice residency faculty and is the volunteer medical director of the Pediatric Mobile Health Clinic sponsored by the Sharp Chula Vista Hospital, which provides care for medically underserved school children in the community.

Dr. Avila is a highly sought speaker on exercise, nutrition, women's health, asthma, preventive medicine, and public health. She has published research in the area of exercise and nutrition for Latina women and was highlighted in *Prevention* magazine. She was most recently featured in an issue of *Ladies' Home Journal* entitled Best of the Best Doctors' Favorite Home Remedies.

Dr. Avila is an avid tennis player, and she has waterskiied since her youth. She also encourages her patients to take walks with her as part of her efforts to put preventive medicine and health promotion into practice.

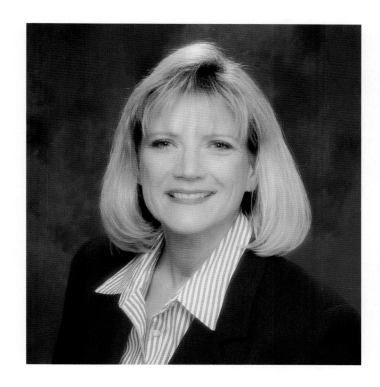

PREFACE

I wrote *Fitness for Health and Sports* to help motivate people to engage in regular physical activity in the pursuit of good health and a feeling of well-being and to promote participation in sports. As a primary care physician serving a large multicultural population in private practice as well as the athletes at the ARCO Olympic Training Center, I have had the unique opportunity and privilege to hear personal stories of staying fit and keeping healthy from people in all walks of life.

But it is the joy, desire, dedication, and spirit of the elite Olympic athletes as they train and compete in the Games that is particularly inspiring. They are the bright exemplars of physical fitness who act as role models for those of us spectators who want to become more physically active or for us weekend warriors who want to perform at a higher level. Throughout this book, their dynamic photos and personal profiles motivate us to exercise and to maintain a higher level of fitness.

To help you achieve those goals, this book offers an integrated and balanced approach to health and fitness that applies to all sports and to all levels of fitness. No matter what your level of fitness may be, or whether you're an exercise contemplator, a weekend warrior, or an elite athlete, this book has something for you. The narrative is organized into four parts. Each part can be read separately or in sequence, depending on your individual needs. *Fitness for Health and Sports* can also be used as a quick-reference guide, so keep this book in a convenient location, and refer back to it whenever you need to. It will also help maintain your motivation to stay fit.

The eye-popping photos in Part I will get your blood moving and start you thinking about your own flexibility, strength, endurance, and fitness.

Part II, Getting Ready, sets optimal health goals and helps you to determine your own personal fitness level. You will learn how to monitor your fitness success through monitoring your heart rate and pulse. Examples are presented on how to overcome exercise barriers such as not having time to exercise. You will also learn how to develop, monitor, and maintain a personal exercise program. Information on body shaping and nutrition rounds out this part.

Part III provides information on how to safely stretch and strengthen your body. We start with your head and work through all the major muscle groups, ending up with your feet. Olympic athletes and trainers demonstrate the various stretches and strengthening exercises. Easy-to-follow directions accompany the photos.

Part IV, Sports Injuries, begins with a discussion about the kinds of injuries related to sports and physical activity, the levels of their severity, and which injuries you can treat yourself, which injuries require professional medical care, and which injuries are emergencies. The narrative then focuses on the various parts of the body individually, starting with the head and neck and proceeding down to the feet. In each section, the muscular and skeletal anatomy is presented first, as a foundation for understanding the probable causes of injuries and how to prevent them. Common injuries are then described, along with procedures for care and rehabilitation. Anatomical drawings and photographs generously illustrate the concepts examined in the narrative. Examples of potential problems are drawn from a wide range of sports, as well as tips for preventing them.

Parts III and IV also feature profiles of Olympic athletes. In Part III, the athletes offer recommendations about stretching and strength training, and in Part IV about injuries they suffered and the process of rehabilitation they went through before returning to the Games. This adds a personal feeling to this book.

The appendixes lay out a Personal Fitness Program and give additional information on a variety of sports medicine topics such as sun protection, heat-related illness, proper sports apparel and shoes, and examples of good nutrition, along with tips on how to maintain your weight. Some appendixes, such as the body weight tables, are quick references. From other appendixes you can photocopy the fitness logs and use them to keep track of monthly progress. In addition, to help maintain your overall health, a chart of preventive medicine guidelines helps you know when to seek screening tests recommended by most leading medical authorities.

Acknowledgments

Developing a book that incorporates detailed narrative, technical and anatomical illustrations, colorful graphics, and dynamic photographs is truly a team effort. This book would not have become a reality without the efforts and support of such a team. It is here that I would like to thank the numerous team members.

First, I would like to thank Hal Lockwood, my editor, who "planted the seed" for the conceptual development of this book, and I am very grateful for his stellar expertise, creative guidance, support, hard work, unending energy, and motivation to carry this project through to completion.

I would like to thank all of my colleagues at the U.S. Olympic Training Centers, particularly Bob Beeten, Director of Sports Medicine, and Jenny Stone, ATC, from the Colorado Springs Olympic Training Center, for their support, recommendations, and guidance throughout this project. Also a special thanks to all of my colleagues at the ARCO Olympic Training Center in Chula Vista, California, for their time, support, numerous phone conversations, photo sessions, and recommendations. I would like to express special appreciation to Vinny Comiskey, ATC, who was always available to give advice and to provide support, and to the athletic trainers: Laureen Selby, Lori Ray, Angela Nava, Chad Forsythe, and

Cheryl Flanders. Thank you also to my physician colleagues, David Flood, M.D., Heinz Hoenecke, Jr., M.D., and Anthony Saglimbeni, M.D.

I would also like to thank all of the athletes mentioned or pictured in the book and anyone I have possibly missed. In particular, I am grateful to Benita Fitzgerald Mosley, Director of the U.S. Olympic Training Centers, for her recommendations, support, and invaluable insights about the Olympic athlete. In addition, many thanks to the United States Olympic Committee and the Public Information and Media Relations Division for supporting this project.

A portion of the profits from this book will be donated to the U.S. Olympic Committee and their SportsMed 2000 fund. SportsMed 2000 is a special program of the Sports Medicine Division dedicated to delivering the best sports medicine care to Olympic athletes and hopefuls, using cutting-edge technology and facilities, and to serving as a center for education in sports medicine.

I am also grateful for the assistance and expertise of Mary Beth Salmon, designer, Trina Stahl, layout artist and compositor, Elizabeth Morales, illustrator, and the photographers Al Bruton, David Knoll, and Scott Gardner. Thank you all. To my typists, Susan Lancaster and Diane Barnes, thank you for taking my handwritten drafts and turning them into a legible manuscript.

I would like to thank my sponsoring editor, Vernon L. Avila, Ph.D., for his review and timely comments about the manuscript, along with the other professionals who reviewed the book's text and illustrations: Julie Moyer Knowles, PT, ATC, Ph.D.; John Lombardo, M.D.; Jenny Stone, ATC; and J. T. Kearney, Ph.D.

Finally, thank you to my family, Vernon, Patrick, and Raquel, for their patience and love throughout this endeavor. Thank you also to my parents and sisters for their kind words of encouragement.

I hope that you enjoy reading this book and that you will apply the health, fitness, and sports concepts to your daily life. Live in good health!

Patricia G. Avila, M.D., M.P.H.

FOREWORD

Every now and then a publication comes along where the parts just seem to flow together. Dr. Patricia Avila's book is one of those. Taken from her experience working with the athletes at the ARCO Training Center, the information comes to you straightforward and factual, and with the use of colorful and interesting graphics, she makes complex ideas easy to understand, so you can hook together your own personalized fitness program. Easy to read, objective, and loaded with good tips on a wide range of health issues, *Fitness for Health and Sports* covers a broad scope of topics designed for better health for a broad population.

The book is written from the perspective of a physician interested in preventive health, where exercise can be simple but integrated into an overall improvement in lifestyle. The American way of diving head first into fitness and trying to accomplish too much too soon is moderated by Dr. Avila into a sense of progression, so that you have an idea of where you can start and how to do it.

Now you can be a winner too. And it can be easy!

Bob Beeten
Director of Sports Medicine
U.S. Olympic Committee

FITNESS

FOR HEALTH AND SPORTS

PART I

The joy of physical

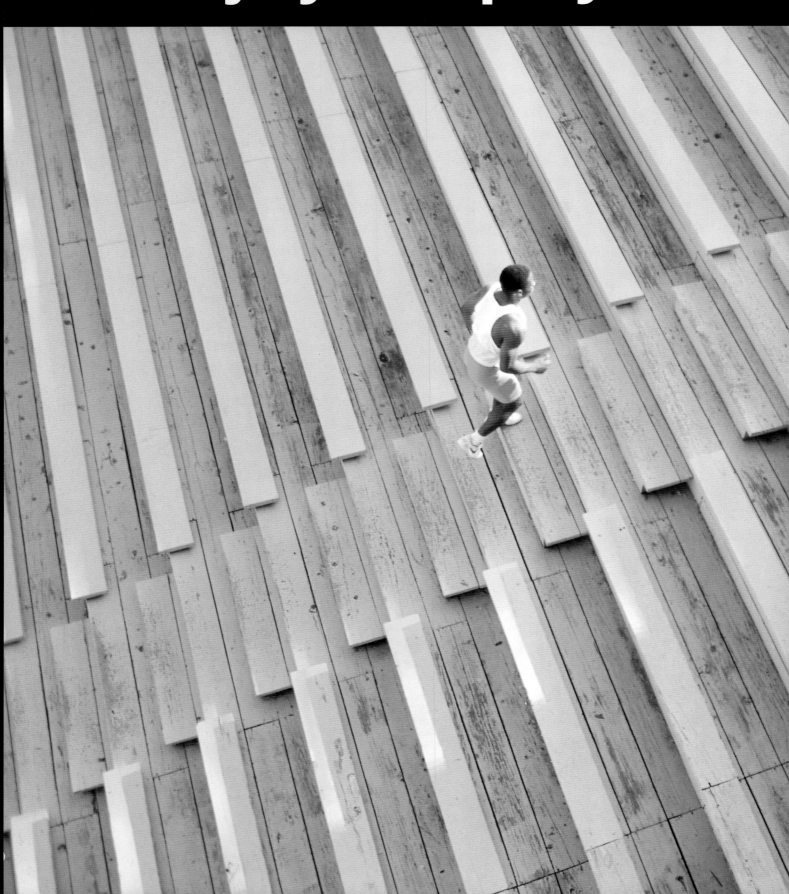

fitness

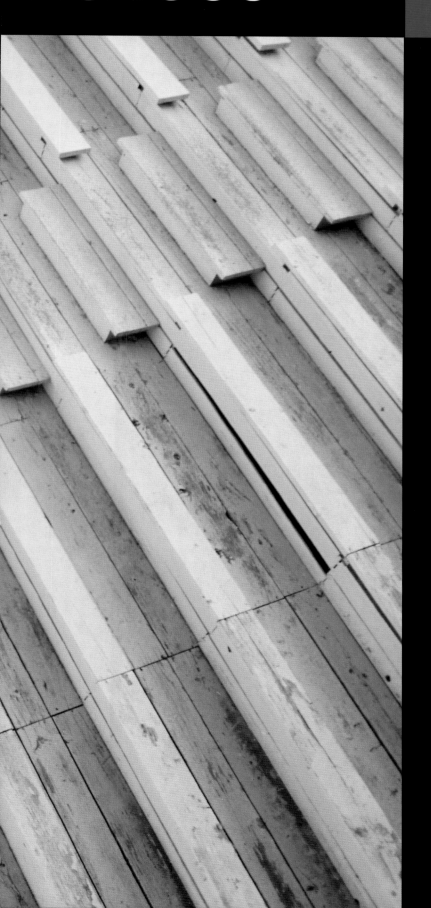

Beauty

Flexibility

Strength

Endurance

Longevity

Camaraderie

Victory!

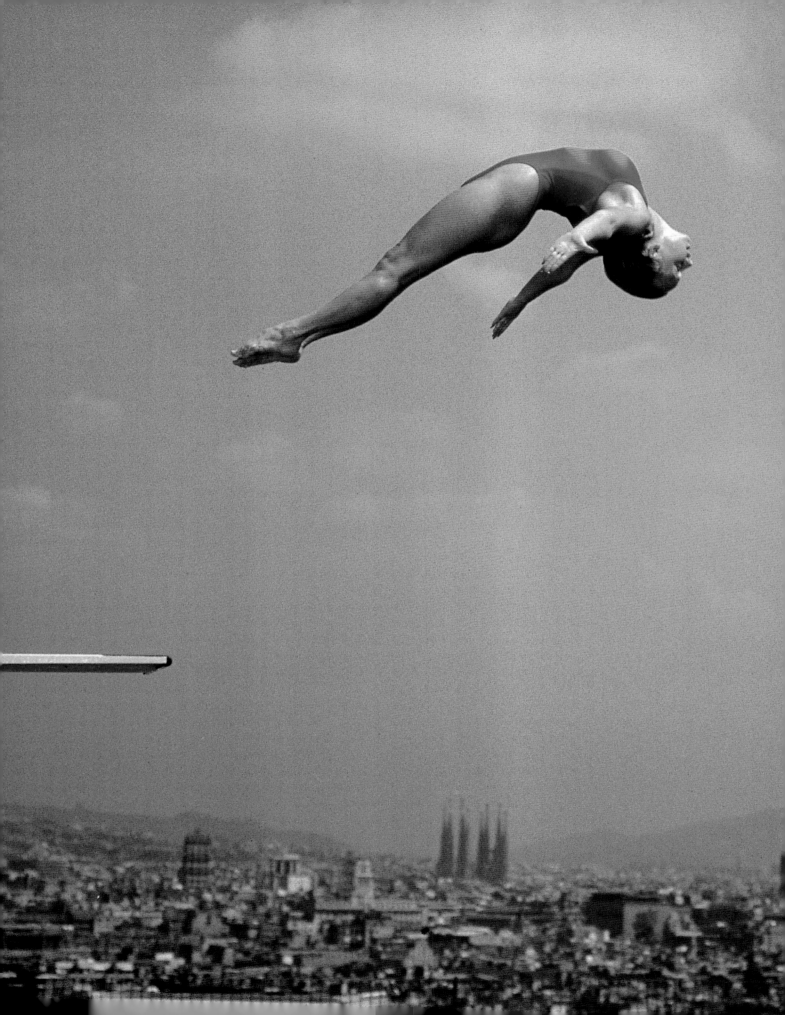

Beauty

The magnificent, taut body of Olympic diver Tracey Mills soaring gracefully above the skyline of Barcelona is a marvel to behold.

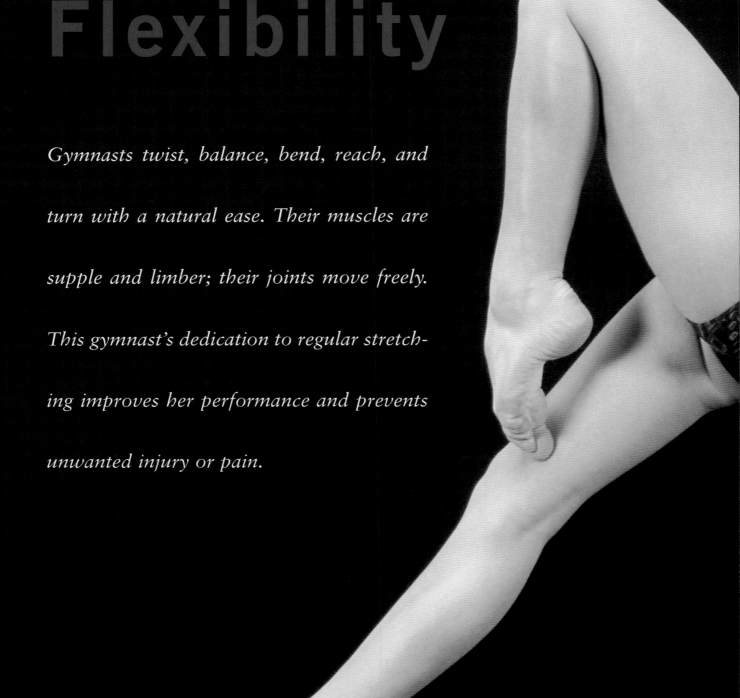

Flexibility

Gymnasts twist, balance, bend, reach, and turn with a natural ease. Their muscles are supple and limber; their joints move freely. This gymnast's dedication to regular stretching improves her performance and prevents unwanted injury or pain.

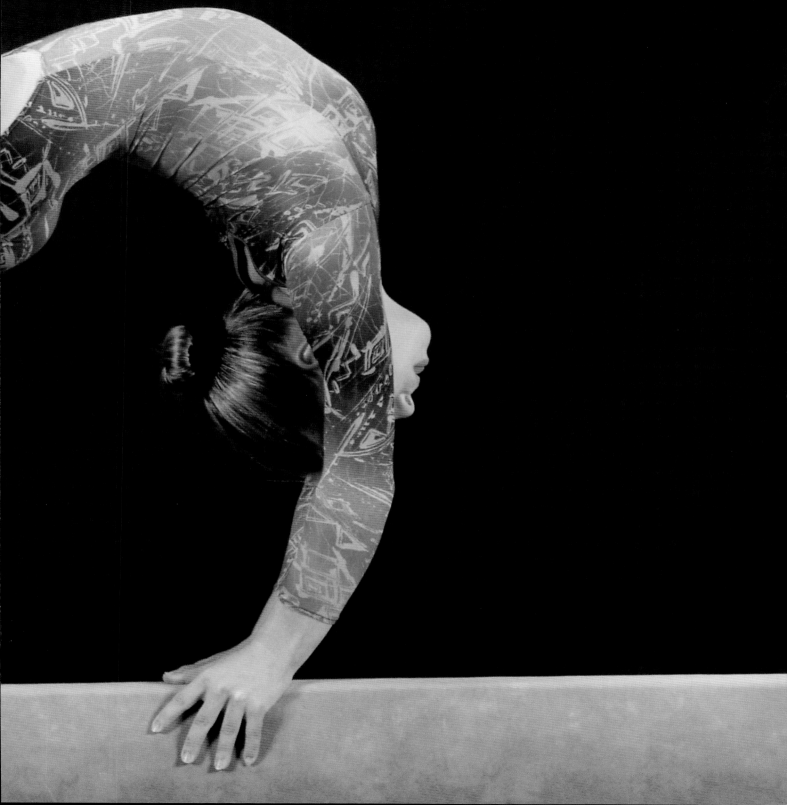

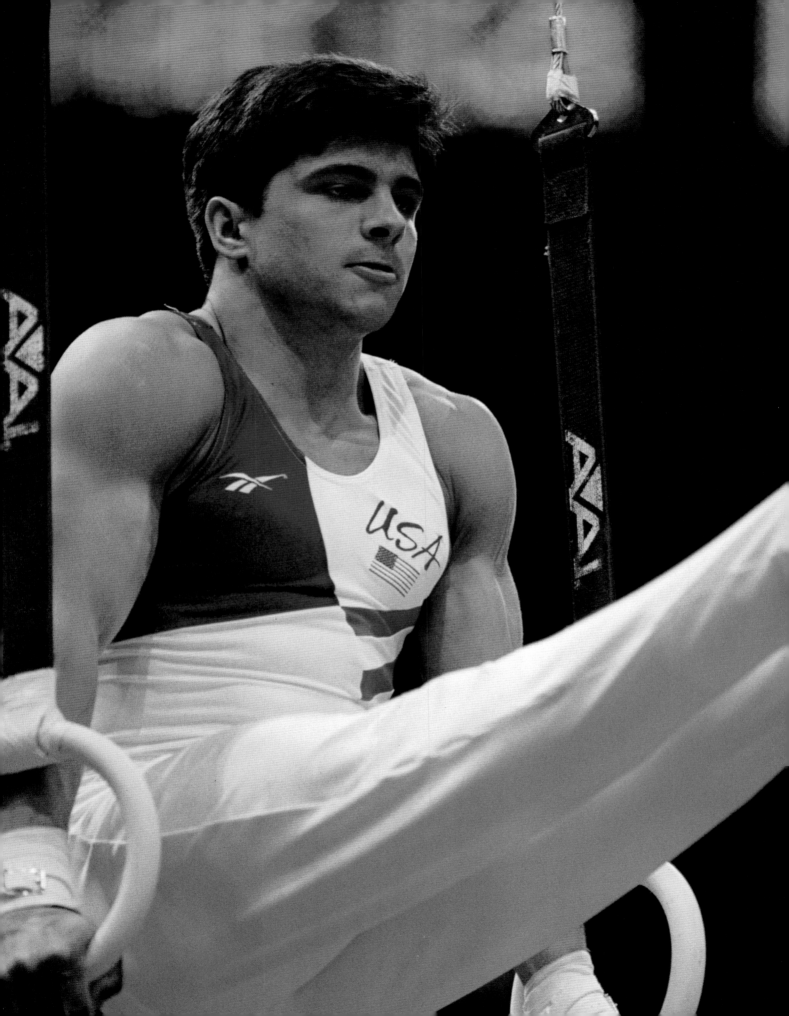

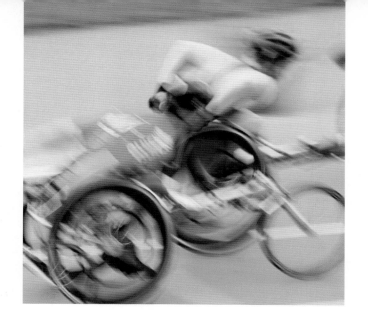

Strength

The triceps muscles contract and bulge as Kip Simons lifts himself seemingly without effort above the rings. Setting his jaw, he raises his legs to a perfect pike position and maintains it, stone still, for three long seconds. Muscular strength is essential to all sports, whether it's the power needed to perform on the rings or to race a wheelchair.

Endurance

Stamina and persistence are winning qualities of distance runners. Dedication and perseverance in daily exercise will improve your endurance whether you are running the 400-meter like Michael Johnson or just trying to keep up with your family.

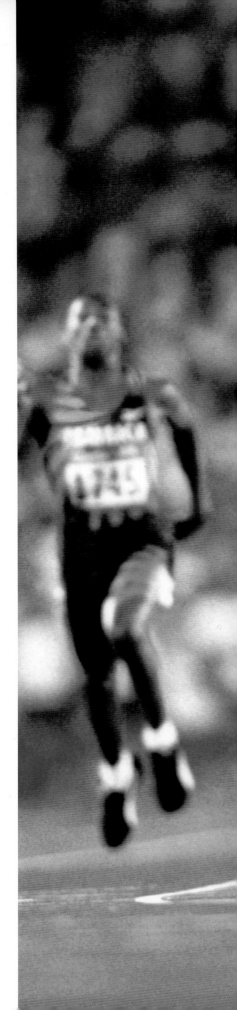

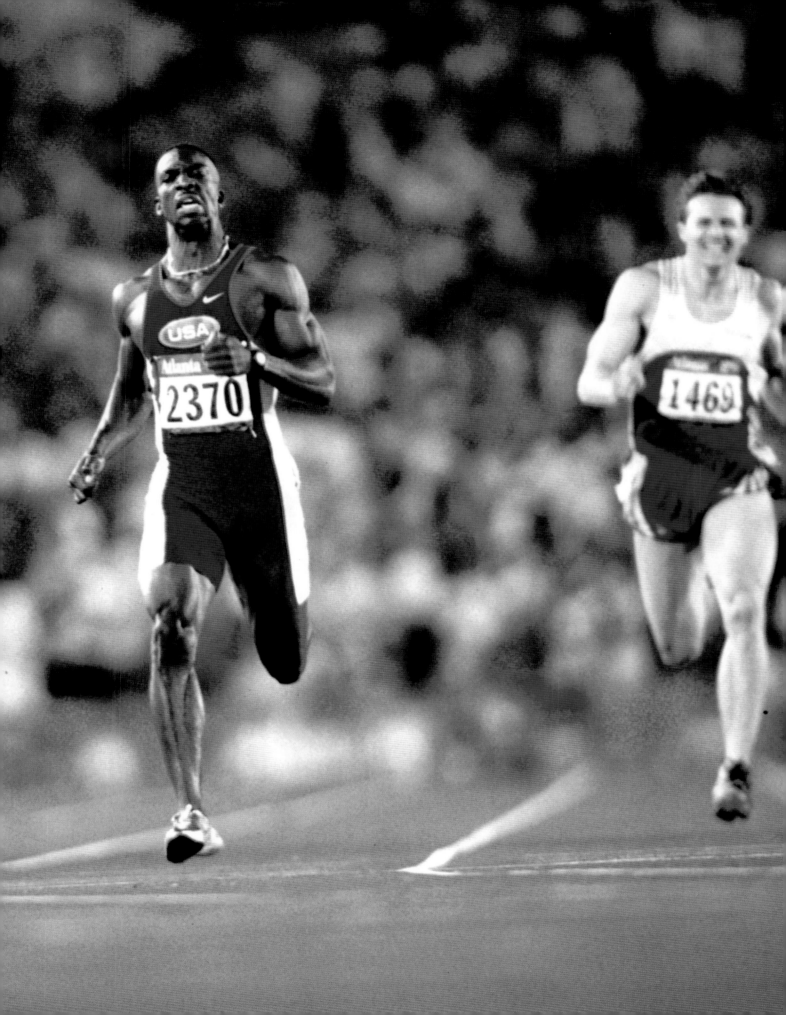

Longevity

An active life filled with moderate activity

should be a positive experience without pain,

denial, or deprivation.

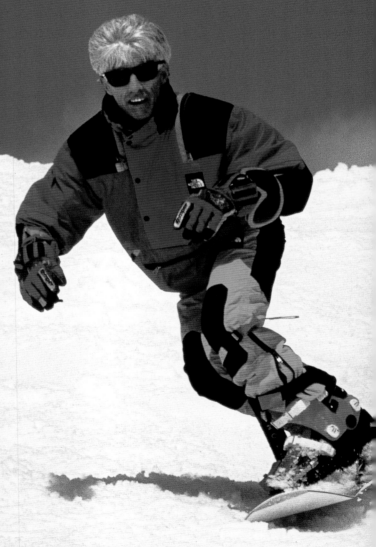

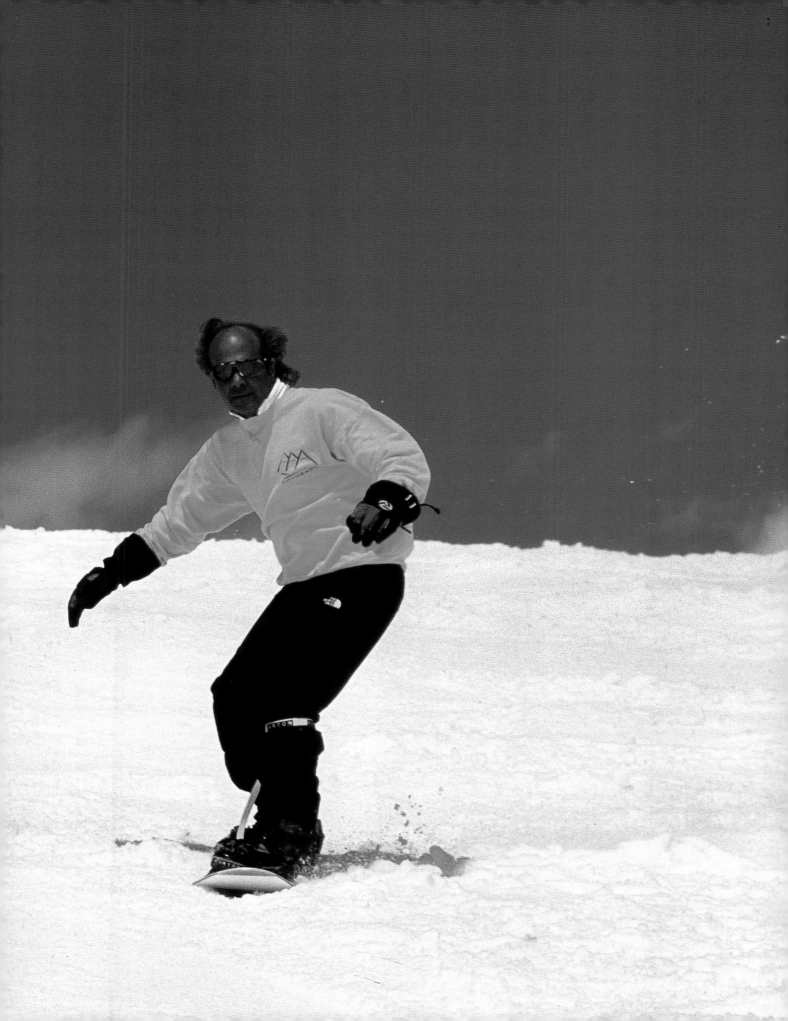

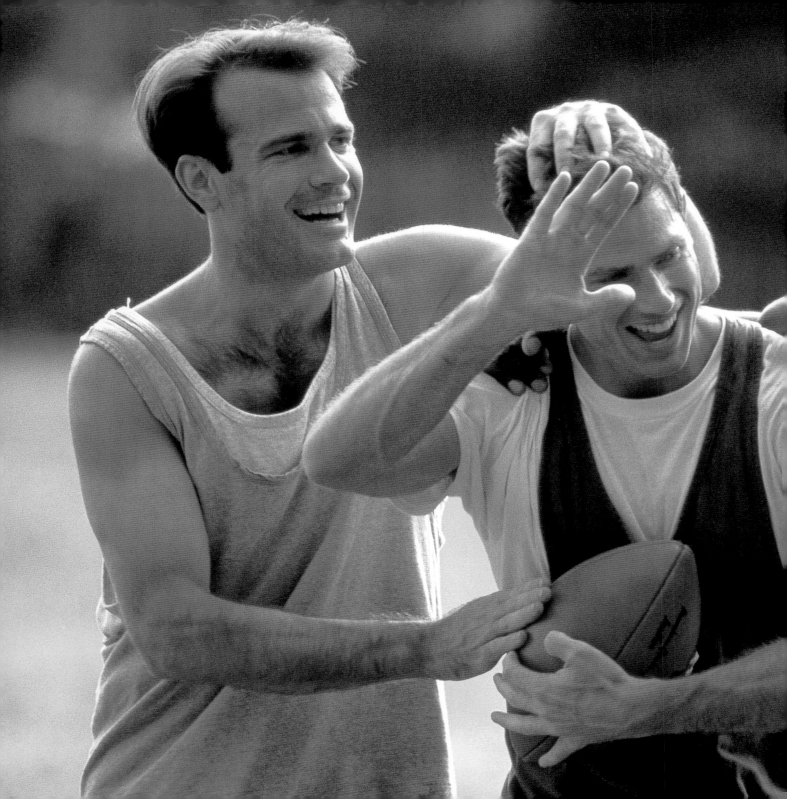

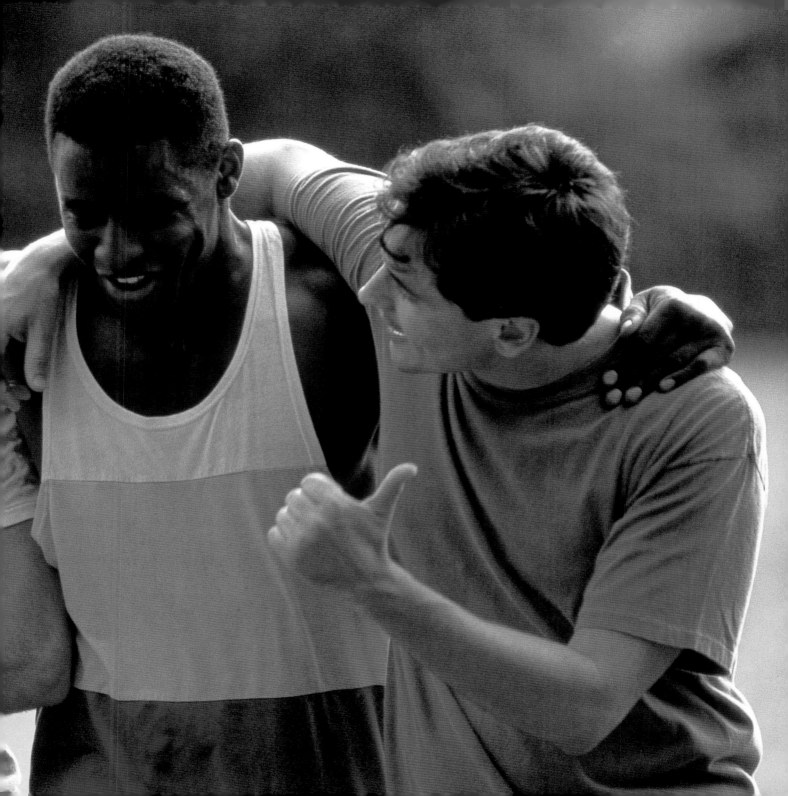

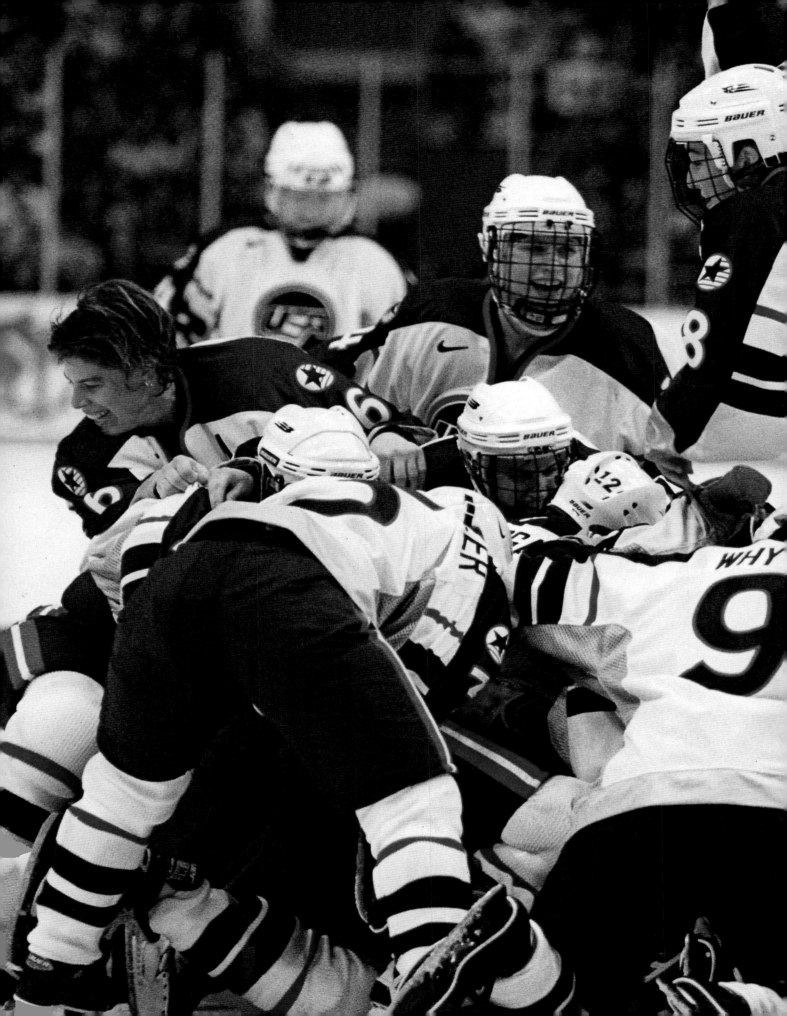

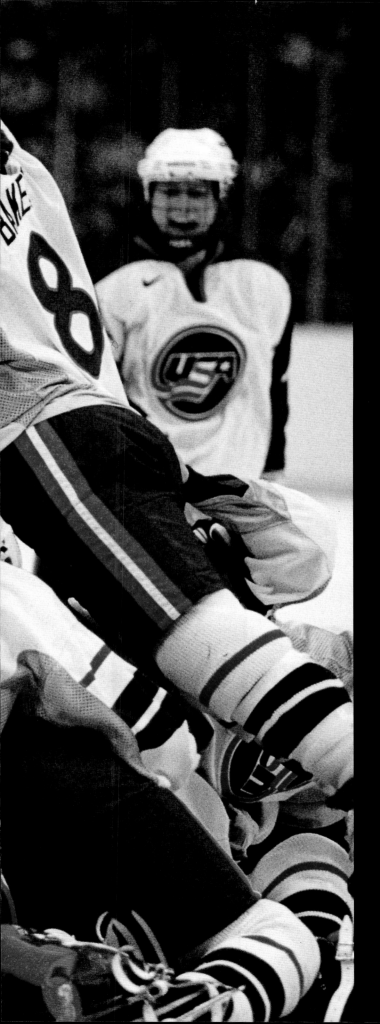

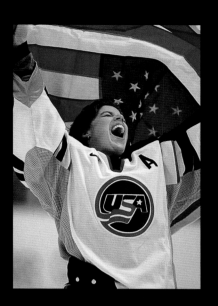

Victory!

We rejoice in the triumph of the human body and spirit, like the Women's Hockey Team winning the gold at Nagano in 1998.

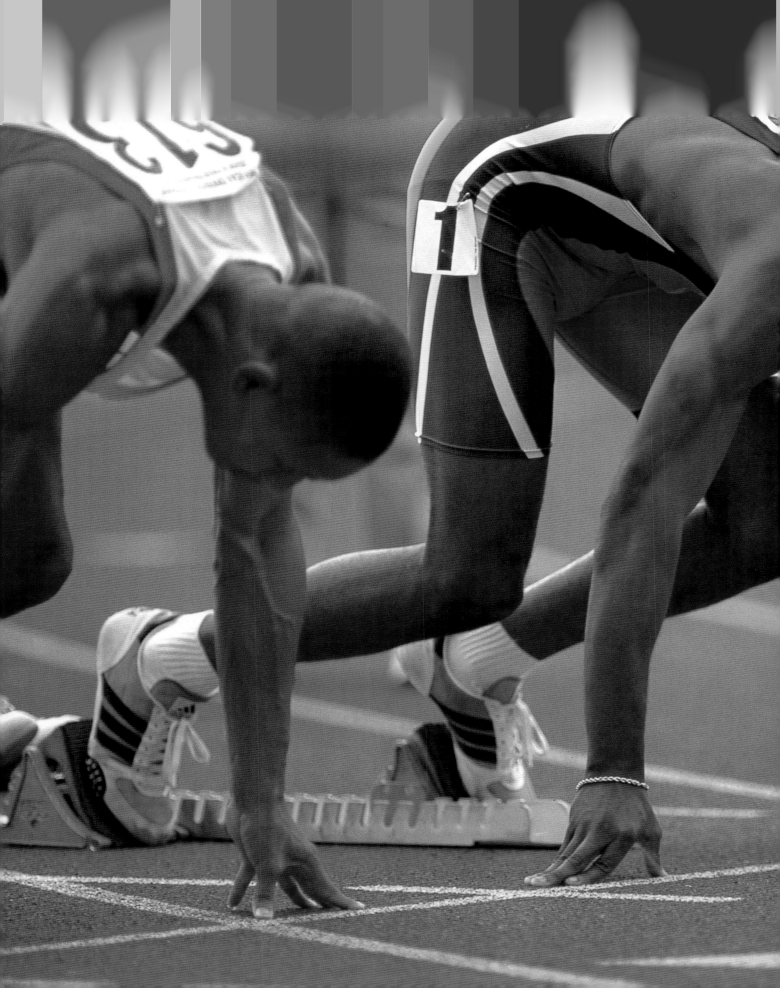

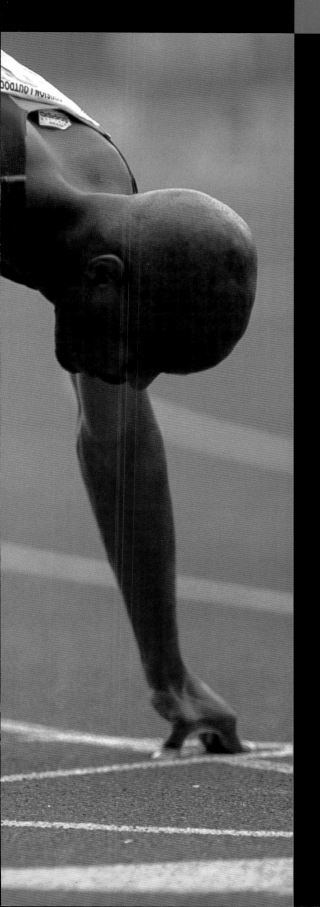

Optimal health

Setting goals

Fitness assessment

Target heart rate

Monitor your heart rate

Aerobic fitness

Aerobic benefits

The FIT program

Muscular fitness

Muscular strength

Muscular endurance

Body shaping

Body composition

The food pyramid

Food choices

A healthy mind and body

Optimal health

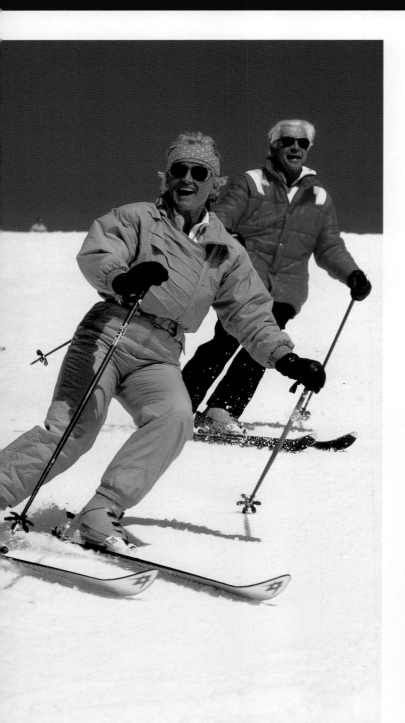

Living a quality life through exercise and proper nutrition yields tremendous health benefits to our physical, mental, and emotional well-being.

Playing it safe

Knowing your own limits and using common sense is important before increasing your activity level. If you haven't been active on a regular basis for over a year, if you are older than 40, or if you answer Yes to any of the following questions, it is advised that you see your medical doctor before beginning your exercise program.

QUESTIONS

- Do you frequently have chest pain?

- Has a doctor ever told you that you have heart disease (or heart problems)?

- Do you have high blood pressure?

- Have you ever felt dizzy or faint?

- Do you have any bone or joint problems?

- Are you over the age of 40 and not accustomed to exercise?

- Do you take any medications?

- Is there any reason, not mentioned here, why you should not follow an exercise program?

Source: Adapted from the British Columbia Department of Health Physical Activity Checklist.

The four components of fitness

AEROBIC FITNESS improves the heart and lungs.

FLEXIBILITY allows you to move your joints freely without pain through a wide range of motion.

MUSCULAR STRENGTH AND ENDURANCE allow your body to work longer before getting tired.

BODY COMPOSITION is vital for maintaining health and preventing chronic illness by keeping normal weight and body measurements.

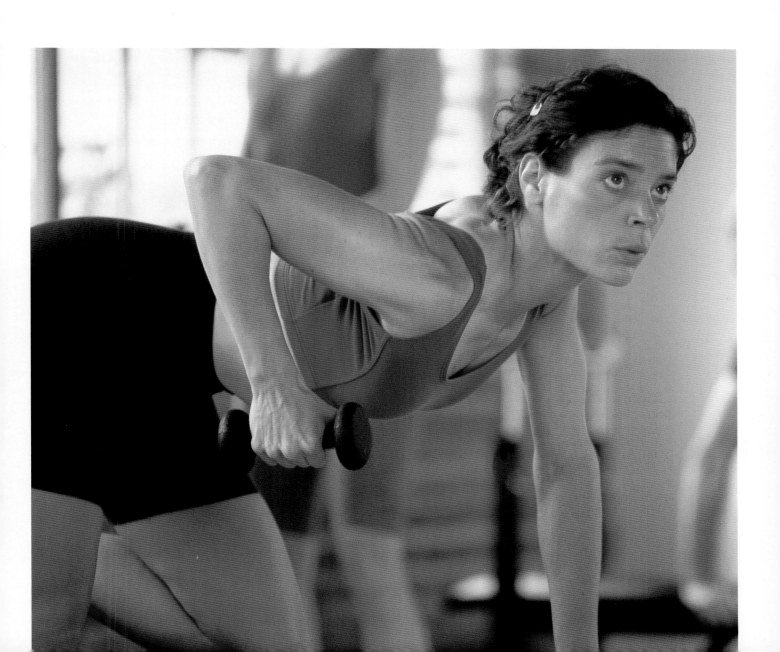

Setting goals

Goals

The American College of Sports Medicine, along with the President's Council on Physical Fitness, recommends that Americans lead more active lifestyles. The minimum goal of all Americans is to have 30 minutes of moderate physical activity over the course of the day most days of the week.

Once you are active, improved fitness is directly related to the frequency of exercise. In other words, the more exercise sessions per week, the more you improve your overall fitness. When your fitness improves, it will be much easier during your exercise sessions to increase the intensity (amount of work) and duration (length of time) of your exercise.

If you prefer more intense and more frequent exercise sessions per week, allow yourself adequate time for recovery. At least one day of rest per week will help prevent overuse injuries and illness due to an overworked immune system.

The same holds for performance. If you

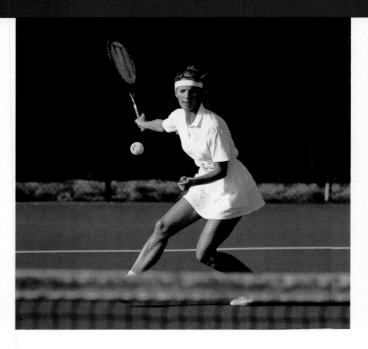

play a particular sport and if you would like to improve your performance, keep in mind that the more time you practice, the better you will become.

What is moderately intense activity?

A wide range of activities can contribute to a moderately intense program of 30+ minutes. This includes everyday activities you already may be doing, such as walking the dog, mowing the lawn, and vacuuming the house, or it can include planned activities such as cycling, swimming, playing tennis, and dancing.

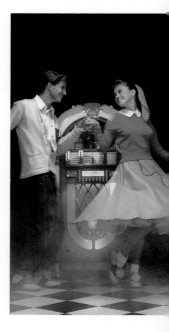

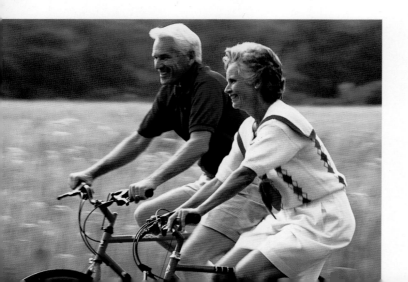

Overcoming hurdles

Everyone faces hurdles to becoming more active. Some are physical, but many are not. Here are some proven solutions to overcoming common obstacles:

Hurdle	Solution
Can't get motivated.	Identify people who are fit, and use them as your role model. Identify a "buddy" who will support you and/or get active with you. Set short-term goals and reward yourself. Do it for yourself and have fun!
No time.	Walk in place while watching television. Set your alarm clock to get up 15 minutes earlier. Use the stairs. Walk at lunch. Walk in place while talking on the telephone. Reset your priorities.
Don't know how to get started.	Increase the amount, frequency, and time of activities that you already do as part of your everyday routine. Walk the dog 15 minutes longer. Use the stairs more than once a day; then increase the number of times you take the stairs. Start off doing more activities slowly, and gradually increase the amount of time spent on your activities every week. Match your type of activity to things you enjoy, such as walking, gardening, hiking, biking, running, dancing, or swimming.
You're physically fit but want to play a particular sport better.	Congratulations on your fitness! However, fitness and athletic performance are two different things. Schedule practice time for your favorite sport three to four times a week in addition to maintaining your fitness program.

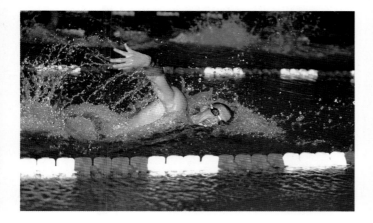

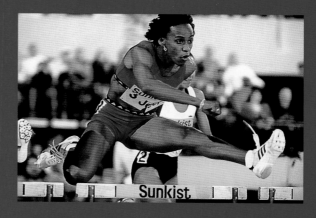

Jackie Joyner-Kersee

Many people have physical challenges to overcome, including some of the top Olympic athletes. Take Olympic gold medalist Jackie Joyner-Kersee, for example. She is well known as the first woman to win consecutive Olympic gold medals (1988 and 1992) in the heptathlon, a grueling two-day competition comprised of the 200-meter dash, 100-meter hurdles, high jump, long jump, shotput, javelin throw, and 800-meter run. And she not only won the event but smashed world records for points scored.

What makes her accomplishment even more extraordinary is that she has exercise-induced asthma, which makes it difficult to breathe. Yet Jackie has stated that by developing a positive mental attitude and by following proper medical advice and treatment she has been able to overcome this health problem. She also believes that maintaining a consistent exercise program makes it much easier. She says, "Even if you're not an athlete, you can still be healthy and active every day."

Fitness assessment

What is your current level of physical fitness? By ascertaining this and your own comfort level, you will avoid unwanted injuries or frustration. Use the following self-survey to determine your current fitness level and how many minutes of continuous activity in each session you should begin with.

Now that you know how long you should work out, the next question is, what level of intensity of physical activity is right for you, in terms of providing safety and giving the most health benefits? To determine this, follow the next steps to calculate your personal Target Heart Rate Zone.

Self-Survey
PHYSICAL ACTIVITY ASSESSMENT

Use the number (0–7) that best describes your general activity level for the previous month.

I do not participate regularly in programmed recreation, sport, or heavy physical activity.

0   Avoid walking or exertion (for example, always use the elevator, drive whenever possible instead of walking).

1   Walk for pleasure, routinely use stairs; occasionally exercise sufficiently to cause heavy breathing or perspiration.

I participate regularly in recreation or work requiring modest physical activity, such as golf, horseback riding, calisthenics, gymnastics, table tennis, bowling, and yard work.

2   10–60 minutes per week.

3   More than 1 hour per week.

I participate regularly in heavy physical exercise, such as running or jogging, swimming, cycling, rowing, skipping rope, running in place, or engaging in vigorous aerobic activity type exercise, such as tennis, basketball, or handball.

4   Run less than 1 mile per week or spend less than 30 minutes per week in comparable physical activity.

5   Run 1–5 miles per week or spend 30–60 minutes per week in comparable physical activity.

6   Run 5–10 miles per week or spend 1–3 hours per week in comparable physical activity.

7   Run more than 10 miles per week or spend 3 hours per week in comparable physical activity.

Assessment

If you rated 0–3, start your exercise program with about 10 minutes of continuous activity each session.

If you rated 4 or above, try to exercise 30 minutes or more each session.

Reprinted, by permission, from R. M. Ross and A. S. Jackson, "The NASA/JSC Assessment of Current Physical Activity," in *Exercise Concepts, Calculations, and Computer Applications* (Dubuque, Iowa: Brown & Benchmark, 1990).

Target heart rate

Your Target Heart Rate Zone is the best way to monitor the intensity of physical activity. The optimal heart rate for exercise lies between 60 percent and 80 percent of the maximum heart rate (or beats per minute) for your age.

The optimal Target Heart Rate Zone for a 40-year-old is calculated as follows:

Maximum heart rate = 220 − 40 = 180
Lower limit exercise heart rate = 180 x 0.60 = 108
Upper limit exercise heart rate = 180 x 0.80 = 144
Target Heart Rate Zone = 108 to 144 beats per minute

Calculate yours with the following formula:

Maximum heart rate (MHR) = 220 − your age = _____
Lower limit exercise heart rate = MHR x 0.60 = _____
Upper limit exercise heart rate = MHR x 0.80 = _____

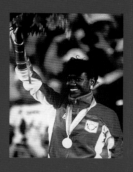

Benita Fitzgerald Mosley

When she won the gold medal in the 100-meter hurdles at the 1984 Olympics, Benita was only the second American and the first African-American woman to win that event. Earlier in her career she was National Champion eight times and an All-American fifteen times. On top of these accomplishments, *Track and Field News* named Benita Fitzgerald Mosley Hurdler of the Decade for the 1980s. Today Benita is Director of the U.S. Olympic Training Centers.

Throughout her life, periodic physical assessment has been important to Benita in continuing her personal fitness plan.

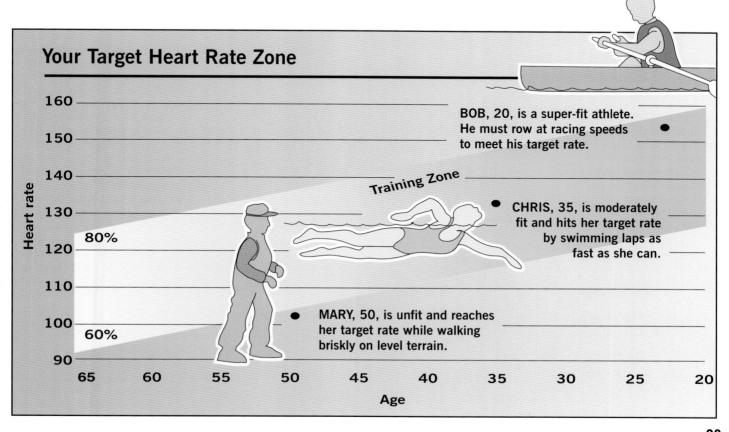

Your Target Heart Rate Zone

Training Zone

BOB, 20, is a super-fit athlete. He must row at racing speeds to meet his target rate.

CHRIS, 35, is moderately fit and hits her target rate by swimming laps as fast as she can.

MARY, 50, is unfit and reaches her target rate while walking briskly on level terrain.

80%

60%

Heart rate: 160, 150, 140, 130, 120, 110, 100, 90

Age: 65, 60, 55, 50, 45, 40, 35, 30, 25, 20

Monitor your heart

Your heart rate is how many times it beats per minute. There are two easy ways to check this yourself: by feeling for the heartbeat at your wrist (radial pulse) or at the sides of your neck (carotid pulse). However, it is recommended that you take your pulse at the wrist to avoid undue risk. Although it occurs rarely, too much pressure on the carotid artery may stimulate a reflex that slows the heart, or may dislodge a buildup of arterial fat, leading to obstruction of blood flow to the brain.

PULSE-READING TECHNIQUE

Locate your pulse at your wrist or at the side of your neck. Count the number of beats (pulses) in 10 seconds. Count the first beat as 0.

Multiply your 10-second count by 6. This is your heart rate per minute. (Hint: Use a watch with a second hand to count your 10-second pulse. The number of beats in 10 seconds x 6 = heart rate.)

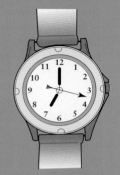

Number of beats in 10 seconds x 6 = Heart rate.

Radial pulse

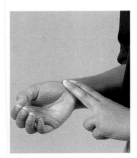

To find the radial pulse, lightly press the pads of your index and middle fingers onto the thumb side of your wrist. Do not use your thumb because it has a pulse of its own.

Carotid pulse

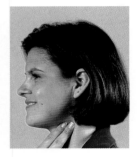

You can also read your heart rate from the pulse in the carotid artery at either side of your neck. Lightly press the pads of your index and middle fingers onto the side of the neck.

Exercise within your Target Heart Rate Zone

As you become more fit, you can safely increase the intensity of your workout. During exercise, monitor your heart rate at various times (for example, after the first 5 or 10 minutes) to adjust your intensity level. As a guide for brisk walking and jogging, use the "talk test": You should be able to carry on a conversation while you exercise. If not, check your heart rate and slow down.

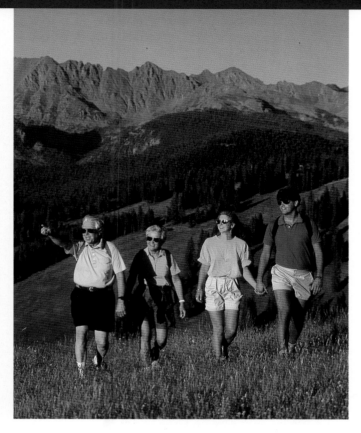

The "talk test."

Your progress in fitness training will be dictated by your commitment to getting active and by your own genetic potential. Physical improvements are most significant or noticeable when you start at a low level of fitness. When you start at a high level, small improvements may not be that noticeable, but maintaining health feels great. If you are highly motivated, you can achieve personal goals with ease. Remember to listen to your body's needs—if you are injured or ill, take time to recover before returning to your exercise program. Excellence in fitness is based on persistence and a well-planned exercise and nutrition program.

Tips for making progress

REST AND SLEEP Adequate rest will increase the gain associated with exercise. Eight or more hours of sleep a night is highly recommended.

NUTRITION Daily intake of a variety of foods, including adequate amounts of carbohydrates and proteins, is essential for fitness. For more nutrition advice, see pages 40–41 and Appendix C.

MATURITY Mature bodies can handle more training than adolescent bodies, because in youth more energy is needed for growth and development.

HEREDITY About 25 percent of fitness is genetically determined. Body type, heart and lung size, height, and other factors are determined by our genes. However, external factors such as diet and exercise influence the expression of our genetic potential.

WATER Drinking eight glasses (8 oz. each) of water a day is important for maintaining cells and body tissue. Water accounts for 60 percent of a man's weight and 50 percent of a woman's weight. If you are physically active you will need to drink more water. Always drink water before, during, and after exercise. If you feel thirsty, your body already lacks water.

Aerobic fitness

Aerobic fitness is endurance, stamina, or the ability to persist in a prolonged endeavor. Aerobic fitness comes from regular, moderate physical activity, which is associated with many health benefits, including some level of protection from heart disease, hypertension, obesity, adult-onset diabetes, and more.

For example, heart disease is associated in some individuals with high levels of blood cholesterol (a fatty substance in foods derived from animal sources, also produced by the liver), which can form deposits on the walls of the arteries (blood vessels that carry blood away from the heart). This can lead to coronary arterial disease (clogged arteries) and eventually heart disease.

One of the primary direct effects of moderate-intensity physical activity is the improved ability of the cardiovascular system (the heart and blood vessels) to mobilize

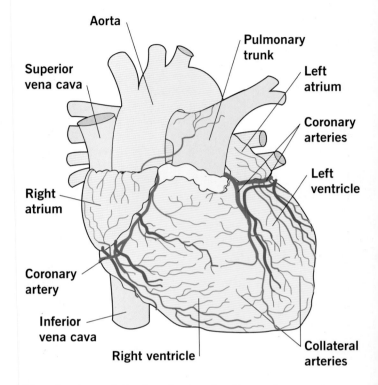

The structure of the heart, showing the major coronary arteries and some collaterals.

and metabolize fat, thereby lowering circulating levels of fat in the blood (triglycerides

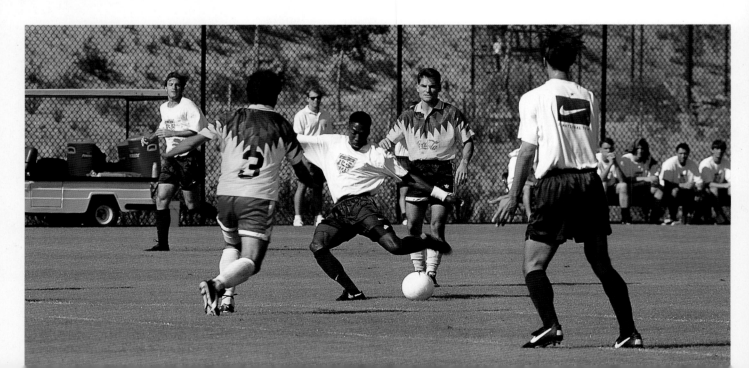

and cholesterol). In addition, moderate physical activity improves circulation within the heart by enhancing the development of alternative circulatory routes (coronary collaterals) that help distribute blood and minimize the effects of narrowed coronary arteries.

Regular physical activity allows your body to adapt to the demands of aerobic exercise. As fitness improves, your heart gets stronger. During exercise, your heart pumps more blood with each beat. The arteries dilate so that more blood (which carries oxygen) can be delivered to your muscles. The muscles of your body adapt by becoming more efficient, absorbing oxygen from the blood and converting carbohydrates, proteins, and fats into energy. In other words, as you become fit you'll be able to exercise and perform other physical activities without running out of energy and feeling tired.

What kind of exercise makes sense?

Choosing aerobic activities that are safe, enjoyable, and effective is key to your overall fitness program. Consider several factors:

CONVENIENCE Some aerobic activities require expensive equipment or traveling. For example, it would be hard to make snow skiing a daily activity if you lived in a tropical climate, or swimming if you had no access to a pool. Choose an activity that is convenient for you and fits your circumstances and resources.

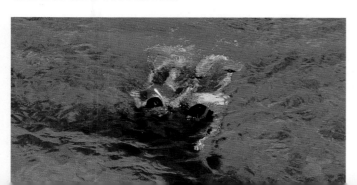

IMPACT Some activities involve jumping or pounding on hard surfaces, which could be uncomfortable or could lead to injury. For that reason, you may want to switch from running or playing basketball to swimming or rowing.

SKILL AND SOCIAL FACTORS Exercising at your own skill level, with people you enjoy, or working out alone and feeling happy are key to maintaining your activity program.

If you've lived a rather sedentary life, starting an exercise program can be hard. By concentrating on simple ways to begin increasing your level of activity, however, you'll be on your way to an enjoyable, active, and fit life. There are many everyday opportunites to do this.

At home

Wash and wax the car
Mow the lawn
Rake the grass or leaves
Shovel snow
Vacuum
Wash windows
Clean the garage
Walk or jog in place while
    watching television

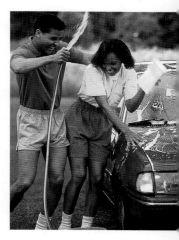

Away from home

Park the car and walk
Fly a kite
Use stairs, avoid elevators
Walk during lunch
Walk down all the aisles in
    the grocery store twice
Bike to work

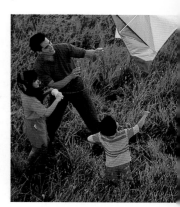

Aerobic benefits

Aerobic exercise improves oxygen intake, transport, and utilization in the heart, lungs, and muscles. It also benefits the nervous and hormonal systems. Aerobic exercise improves the condition and efficiency of your breathing muscles, allowing for greater use of your lung capacity.

In the aerobically fit individual, fewer breaths are needed to move the same volume of air into the lungs. The amount of air moving into and out of your lungs is called ventilation. Ventilation is slower and breaths are deeper, allowing more of each breath to reach the portion of the lungs where oxygen is delivered to the bloodstream and carbon dioxide is released from the bloodstream. This exchange of oxygen and carbon dioxide gas depends on

good ventilation and adequate blood flow to and from the lungs.

The respiratory tract is a system of passageways that lead from the nose and

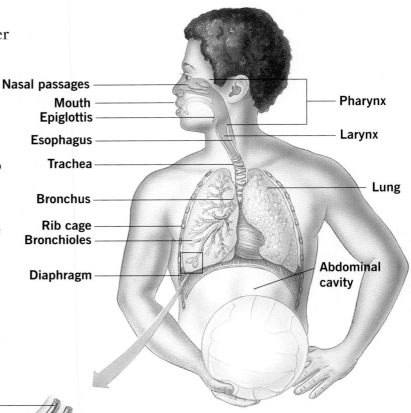

The major organs of the human respiratory system. The function of the respiratory system is the exchange of oxygen and carbon dioxide gases. The photograph at right shows a microscopic view of the alveoli and capillaries.

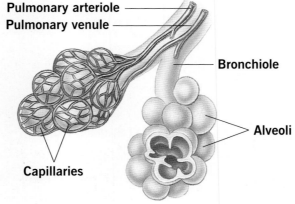

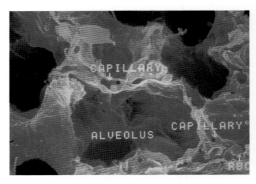

28

mouth to tiny chambers in the lungs called alveoli. The actual exchange of oxygen and carbon dioxide takes place in the alveoli, the air sacs clustered at the end of each bronchiole, or air passage. A tiny blood vessel called a pulmonary arteriole carries deoxygenated blood to the capillaries of

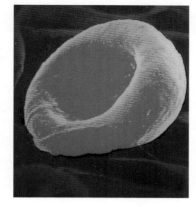

Red blood cells distribute oxygen to the body.

the alveolar sac; a pulmonary venule carries oxgenated blood away from the sac to the rest of the body by the pumping action of the circulatory system (the heart and blood vessels).

Oxygen is transported in the body by the red blood cells (specifically, the hemoglobin of the red blood cells) in the blood. Aerobic fitness increases total hemoglobin levels, thereby making more oxygen available to the body and muscles. Muscles can then utilize oxygen in the breakdown of carbohydrates and fats to produce energy for muscle contraction. Thus aerobic exercise increases the efficiency of the exercising muscles by enabling the muscles to utilize oxygen better.

In addition, the efficient, trained heart (by aerobic activity) pumps more blood each time it beats, at rest or during exercise. The trained heart beats at a slower rate, pumping a larger volume of blood with more oxygen each time it beats. Aerobic fitness improves the ability of the lungs and heart to distribute oxygen throughout the body.

BENEFITS OF AEROBIC FITNESS

- Improves the efficiency of respiration by improving the condition and efficiency of breathing muscles

- Improves blood volume, distribution, and delivery

- Improves cardiovascular efficiency, increasing the amount of blood pumped with each beat of the heart while at the same time lowering the heart rate at rest or during exercise

- Improves the muscles' ability to utilize oxygen, thereby using carbohydrates and fats as a source of energy

- Improves body composition by decreasing body fat relative to lean weight

- Fine tunes the nervous and hormonal systems

- Improves the response of bones, ligaments, and tendons to stress

- Improves psychological outlook and mental functioning

Dan O'Brien, "World's Greatest Athlete."

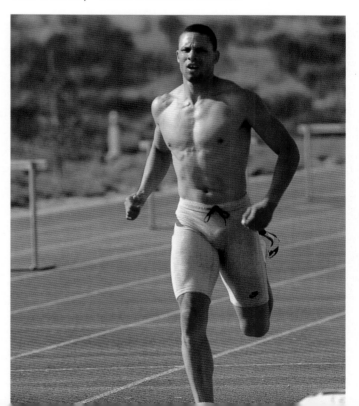

The FIT program

Achieving fitness depends on three factors, represented by the acronym FIT:

Frequency: Most days of the week.
Intensity: Moderate level, using the Target Heart Rate Zone.
Time: Duration of 30 minutes.

If you follow this FIT approach, you will realize all the health benefits generally associated with more intense exercise programs. Keep in mind that it isn't necessary to improve fitness to a high level in order to be healthy and fit. However, you may desire at some point to increase your fitness. You can do this by stepping up the F, I, or T variables. For example, an endurance athlete, such as a long-distance runner, might increase his training time and intensity to perform better in races. You can do the same thing with your program, whether you walk, swim, bike, row, or play tennis. The following example will give you some ideas how to adjust your activity.

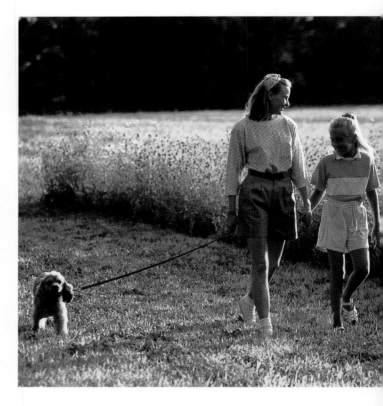

WALKING PROGRAM If you can walk for 10 minutes at moderate intensity, then you are ready to advance to a more intense walking program.

Monday: Walk and extend your walking time by 15 minutes (45 minutes total).

Tuesday: Walk with a brisk stride, using Monday's walking time (45 minutes).

Wednesday: Walk up a hill or stairs for 30 minutes.

Thursday: Walk at intervals: briskly for 15 minutes, then 15 minutes up a hill or stairs (30 minutes total).

Friday: Walk slowly for a long distance (60 minutes total).

Saturday: Hike over varied terrain at a leisurely pace.

Sunday: Rest!

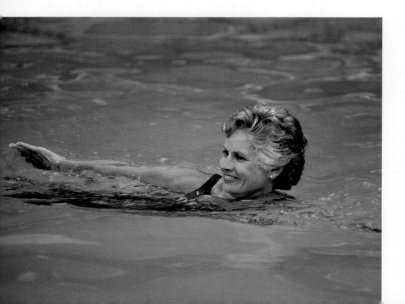

Guidelines for aerobic training

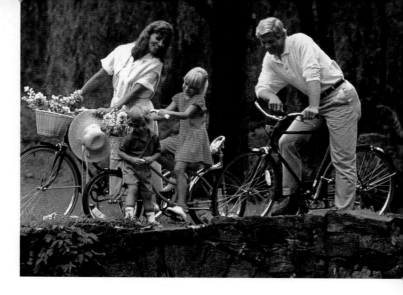

➤ Warm up for at least 5 minutes. A warm-up should always precede an exercise activity to guard against muscle, ligament, and tendon strain. The warm-up should consist of stretching, calisthenics, and a gradual increase in activity before beginning intense exercising. If time permits, take more time, and remember to restretch all major muscle groups (see Part III, pages 46–57).

➤ Exercise for a minimum of 30 minutes most days of the week.

➤ Cool down for at least 5 minutes. A cool-down is just as important as a warm-up. Abruptly stopping a vigorous activity can contribute to cramping and soreness or make the heart more subject to irregular beats. In addition, the cool-down helps lower body temperature and remove metabolic wastes that build up during exercise. If time permits, take more time, and remember to restretch all major muscle groups.

➤ If weight loss is a goal, slowly increase the duration and frequency of your exercise until you feel ready to increase the intensity (always check your Target Heart Rate Zone).

➤ Drink plenty of water during exercise. If you feel thirsty, you already need water. A minimum of eight (8-oz.) glasses of water is recommended daily.

➤ Wear comfortable shoes and clothes (see Appendix F).

➤ Be smart: Protect yourself from over-exposure to sun, wind, cold, and heat.

The Aerobic Training Cycle

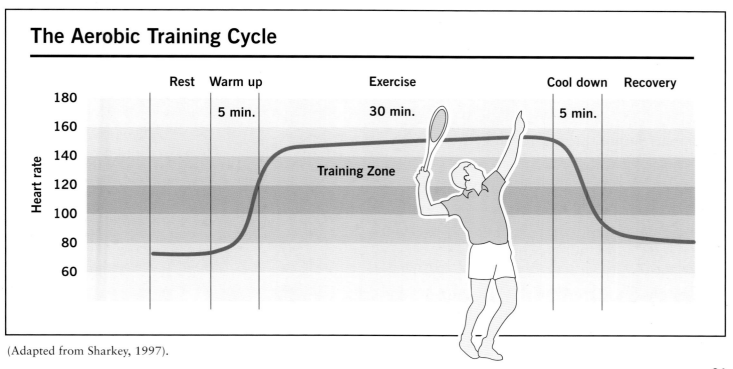

(Adapted from Sharkey, 1997).

Muscular fitness

Everyone would like to have improved strength, muscular endurance, flexibility, speed, power, agility, balance, and coordination. In sports, muscular fitness improves performance in all these ways. But throughout life we need muscular strength to avoid injuries and to participate independently and fully in all sorts of daily activities. It takes strength to mow a lawn, shovel snow, push a vacuum, or carry infants. Increased activity leads to stronger muscles, and stronger muscles lead to a more active life and less fatigue.

Muscular fitness also confers other benefits. For example, abdominal strength training can prevent or help relieve low back problems. General muscular fitness can also help metabolize fat more efficiently and prevent or slow down osteoporosis (bone loss).

Using a combination of strength training exercises (see pages 58–69) to work all major muscle groups is the best way to enhance overall muscular strength. Major muscle groups of the extremities are *antagonistic,* meaning they are arranged in opposing pairs, each pulling in a different direction. As one contracts (shortens), the other relaxes (lengthens), producing smooth, coordinated movements. As an example, let's take a look at the muscles of the upper arms.

When you bend your arm, the *biceps brachii* contracts, pulling the lower arm bones (radius and ulna) up, and the *triceps* muscle relaxes. When you straighten your arm, the triceps contracts, pulling the lower arm bones down, and the biceps relaxes.

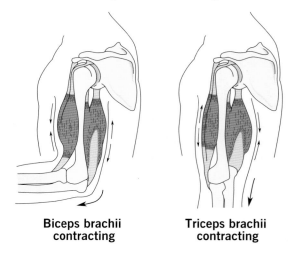

Biceps brachii contracting   **Triceps brachii contracting**

Antagonistic muscles at work.

Muscles that attach to bone (called skeletal muscles) pull on tendons, which in turn pull on and move the bones. Most skeletal muscles are attached to two different bones across a joint. The muscle *origin* is attached to the nonmovable bone during

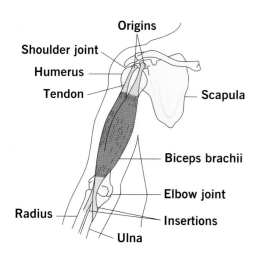

Points of origin and insertion of a skeletal muscle.

contraction, and the muscle *insertion* is the end of the muscle attached to the movable bone. The biceps, for example, originates in the shoulder blade, crosses the elbow joint, and inserts on the bones of the lower arms.

When lifting weights, *flexor* muscles like the biceps decrease the angle of the joint, whereas *extensor* muscles like the triceps increase the joint angle. Flexor and extensor muscles are located in the arm, wrist, hip, leg, and ankle. Muscles that bring limbs to the center of the body—for example, your shoulder girdle—are called *adductors,* and muscles that move limbs away from the center of the body are called *abductors*.

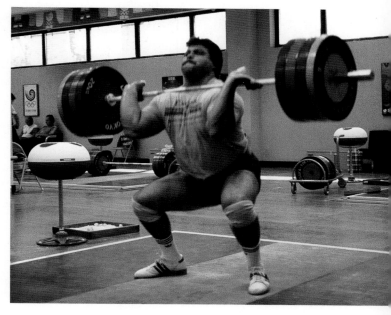

Olympic weightlifter Mario Martinez in training.

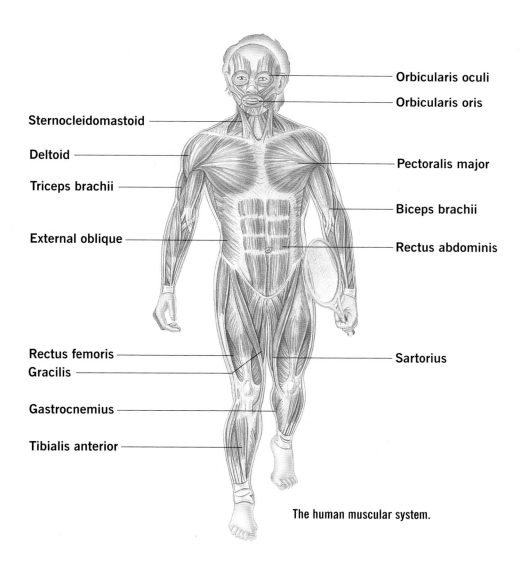

Orbicularis oculi

Orbicularis oris

Sternocleidomastoid

Deltoid

Triceps brachii

Pectoralis major

Biceps brachii

External oblique

Rectus abdominis

Rectus femoris

Gracilis

Sartorius

Gastrocnemius

Tibialis anterior

The human muscular system.

33

Muscular strength

Muscle contraction

Muscle contraction is a dynamic process. Muscles convert chemical energy into mechanical energy for movement. Muscle contraction is dependent on oxygen, chemical energy, and calcium ions. If not enough oxygen is present, lactic acid (another chemical in muscle physiology) can aid the muscle in producing energy for contraction, but only for a short period of time.

Lactic acid can build up in muscles, causing muscular fatigue and soreness. Getting rest and replacing fluids, electrolytes, and oxygen will help with muscular fatigue and soreness. Massaging the muscle will also help to bring oxygen to the muscle, thereby decreasing soreness.

Forget the notion "No pain, no gain"!

If you overdo strength training exercises or improperly do any activity, soreness may result, but it may be delayed for 24 hours. Is this soreness due to lactic acid buildup? Probably not. More likely it is due to slight muscle injury, such as a small tear in the muscle fiber or tendon, or to uncontrolled spasms or contractions of individual muscle fibers because of damage or metabolic byproducts. Rest helps reduce muscle soreness (see pages 76–81 for care of muscle strain and common soft tissue injuries).

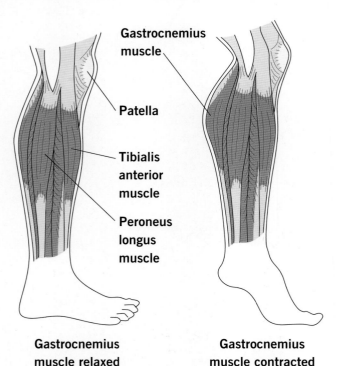

Gastrocnemius muscle

Patella

Tibialis anterior muscle

Peroneus longus muscle

Gastrocnemius muscle relaxed

Gastrocnemius muscle contracted

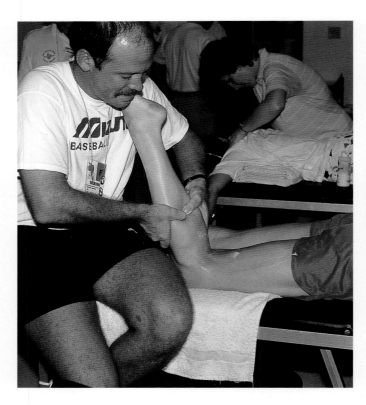

When lactic acid builds up in a muscle like the calf (left), it can cause fatigue. Massaging the muscle (above) brings relief.

How to build muscular strength

Muscular fitness doesn't have to take a lot of time. Two to three short weekly sessions will help you achieve health benefits and reach your goals. For muscle fitness training, you can use simple calisthenics, free weights, or weight machines if they are readily available. Before working with any equipment, make sure you seek advice from a trained instructor. If you are over 40 years of age or have any medical problems, it is recommended that you seek advice from your medical doctor before starting your activity program.

> Muscular strength is the maximal force
> that can be exerted in a
> single voluntary muscle contraction.

Start by training the muscles you would like to improve. The key is to place the muscle under tension (at least two-thirds of maximal strength) by performing several repetitions. Always stretch slowly and warm the muscles before strength training to reduce the risk of injury, and after exercise, cool down the muscles with slow stretches.

For beginners, two to ten repetitions of each exercise in two to three sets is adequate. Working the targeted muscles every other day is all you need. As you become stronger, you can lift more weight and/or increase the number of sets or repetitions. Refer to the strength-training exercises on page 58–69.

Guidelines for **safe** strength training

➤ Always warm up for 5 minutes before exercise and cool down for 5 minutes afterwards.

➤ Muscular fitness is only part of total fitness. Always include a well-planned aerobic program.

➤ Ease into your program. Start with calisthenics, or use lighter weights or resistant rubber bands and do fewer sets if you are a beginner.

➤ Avoid holding your breath during a lift. Exhale during the lift and inhale as you lower the weight.

➤ When lifting free weights, always have a companion "spot" you to avoid problems.

➤ During your workout, alternate major muscle groups.

➤ Allow a few minutes of rest and take sips of water between sets of the same exercise.

➤ Keep a record of your progress (see Appendix A) and always seek expert advice if you have questions.

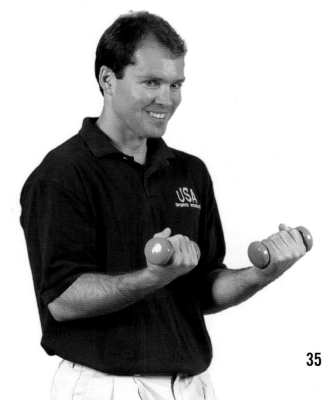

Muscular endurance

Do you have the strength to lift a 10-pound bag of potatoes? Probably so, but how long can you hold up that 10-pound bag before getting tired? In other words, with good muscular endurance you can exercise longer without getting fatigued.

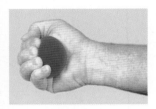
Ball squeeze exercise

The good news is that muscular endurance is trainable. When you have sufficient strength for a particular task, gains in endurance can come with ease. The main difference between training for strength and training for endurance is the level of tension in the muscle, or muscle resistance, and the repetitions. The number of repetitions for endurance training depends on several factors. What are you training for? Is it for short-term or long-term endurance? The following chart will help you plan weight training that fits your goals:

Shoulder/back exercise

Desired effect	Train with
Improved strength	More weight Fewer repetitions
Improved short-term endurance (less than 2 minutes)	Medium weight Medium repetitions
Improved long-term endurance	Less weight (less than 60 percent of maximum strength) More repetitions

Endurance and nutrition

It is important to remember that energy for endurance not only comes from consistent training but from a well-balanced diet. Eating a variety of foods throughout the day, along with adequate amounts of water and carbohydrates, is essential for endurance training. Carbohydrates include whole wheat bread, pasta, cereal, and rice, for example. Without a well-balanced diet of carbohydrates, proteins, and fats, inadequate fuel would be available for the muscles during activities that require endurance. Refer to the food pyramid and guide to daily food choices on pages 40–46.

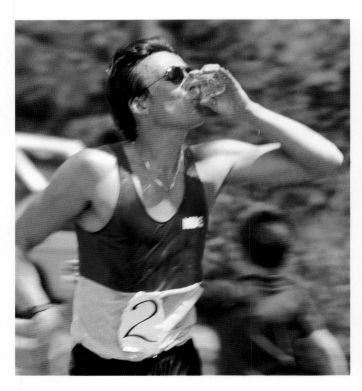
Remember to keep drinking water to maintain your stamina, like runner Adam Goucher.

Body shaping

Weight control and energy balance

By changing the amount and kind of food you eat and the physical exercise you do, you change your energy input and output and your body composition. We talk about this energy in terms of the number of food Calories* consumed and activity Calories expended. For example, if you stayed in bed for 24 hours and did nothing at all, you would expend about 1,600 Calories (for a 154-pound person). The body's energy is used by the lungs for breathing, the heart for pumping blood, the muscles for maintenance, and the body thermostat for temperature regulation. You can increase the energy consumed in this example by simply taking a brisk walk, which burns 5 Calories per minute, or by running, which burns more than 15 Calories per minute.

> Did you know that 1 pound of body fat has the energy equivalent of 3,500 Calories and that 3,500 Calories must be burned through exercise to remove 1 pound of stored fat? Similarly, 3,500 Calories of excess dietary intake will lead to an increase of an additional pound of body weight.

*A Calorie (with a capital C) is defined as the amount of heat energy required to raise 1,000 grams of water (1 liter) one degree Celsius. The daily diet of an average person usually contains 2,000–3,000 Calories of energy.

The key point is that even though proper nutrition will help you maintain your ideal weight, only by getting physical activity can you maintain a "healthy" balance.

Calculating your energy balance

You can learn how to determine your energy balance by calculating your daily caloric food intake and energy output. Maintaining a healthy body composition can be easy. The basic rule of thumb is to participate in daily moderate activity, such as a brisk 30-minute walk, and to eat sensibly.

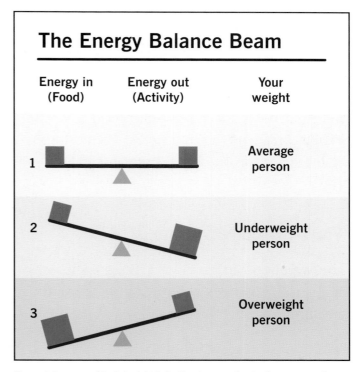

The Energy Balance Beam

Energy in (Food)	Energy out (Activity)	Your weight
1		Average person
2		Underweight person
3		Overweight person

The maintenance of body weight is in direct proportion to the amount of energy taken in as food and the amount of energy output as physical activity. In example 1, the amount of energy taken in equals the amount of energy output, so body weight remains stable. In example 2, low food intake with high physical activity leads to weight loss. In example 3, high food intake with low physical activity leads to increased weight.

Body composition

Physical activity and nutrition are the keys to controlling your body composition. By just keeping your body in motion, such as walking briskly for 30 minutes a day, doing resistance exercises to build lean muscles, and following a well-balanced, low-fat diet, you can keep your weight within desirable limits.

You might say, "I weigh the same as I did when I was 20 years old; I'm not overweight." However, although your weight may be the same, the ratio of lean to fat tissue may not be. Have your waist and hip measurements stayed the same? Did you know that the location of stored fat predicts health risk? A "pot belly" is fat stored in the abdomen and surrounds visceral organs such as the liver, and it is considered a risk factor for heart disease, high blood pressure, stroke, and some cancers.* A "pear shape," or fat stored in the hips, buttocks, and thighs, is not.

Waist-to-hip ratio

The waist-to-hip ratio (WHR) is a measurement used to check whether you are within safe limits.

*Take Note: Gaining more than 10 pounds in early to middle adult life can increase health risks for certain illnesses such as heart disease, high blood pressure, and diabetes.

MEASURING THE WAIST-TO-HIP RATIO Use a soft, flexible tape measure. Measure to the nearest quarter inch. Measure the waist at the navel and the hips at the greatest circumference of the buttocks.

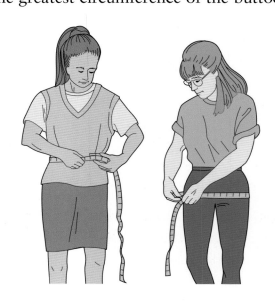

CALCULATING THE WAIST-TO-HIP RATIO Divide your waist measurement by your hip measurement. In this example, the waist measurement (32 inches) divided by the hip measurement (37 inches) = 0.86.

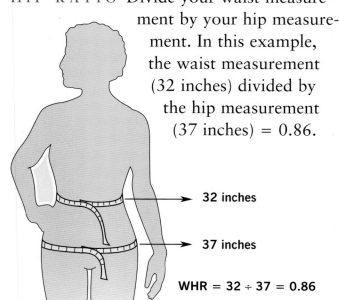

32 inches

37 inches

WHR = 32 ÷ 37 = 0.86

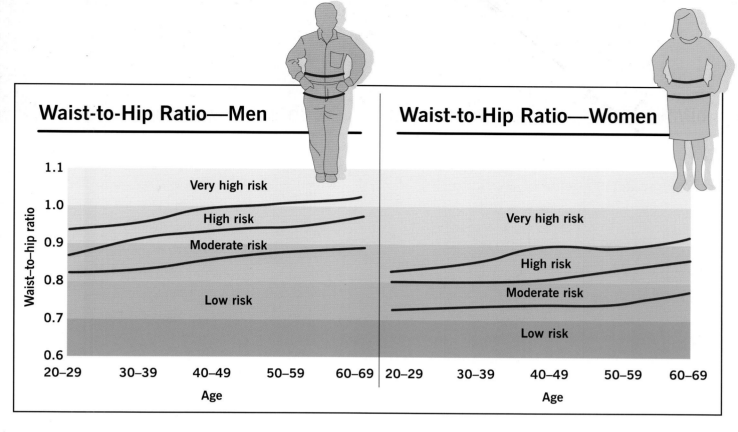

Waist-to-Hip Ratio—Men

Waist-to-Hip Ratio—Women

Waist-to-hip ratio health risks for men and women. (Reprinted by permission of *The Western Journal of Medicine* [G. A. Bray and D. S. Gray, "Obesity: Part I—Pathogenesis" 149 (1988): 429–441]).

WHR SAFE LIMITS The graphs above chart the risk factors associated with different WHR values. People above the upper limits of the WHR range are at high risk for future health problems. Relative safe limits for WHR are the following:

Men = 0.85 to 0.90   Women = 0.75 to 0.80

Other methods to measure body fat such as skinfold measurement, underwater body weighing, and bioelectric impedance require equipment and expert assistance and will not be reviewed here.

Determining healthy weight

Various tables, such as the Body Mass Index, list weights considered to be healthy for women and men of different heights (see Appendix B). Another quick way to calculate your ideal weight is to use the following formulas (estimated weights are plus or minus 10 percent):*

For women: 100 pounds for the first 5 feet, plus 5 pounds for each additional inch
Example: A woman 5 feet 5 inches tall = 100 + (5 X 5) = 125 pounds

For men: 106 pounds for the first 5 feet, plus 6 pounds for each additional inch
Example: A man 5 feet 8 inches tall = 106 + (8 X 6) = 154 pounds

*From Manson et al., 1995.

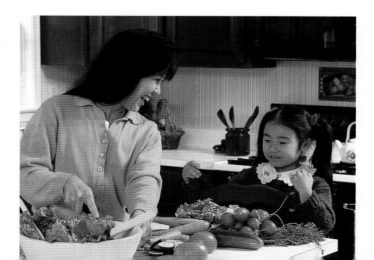

The food pyramid

The U.S. Departments of Agriculture and Health and Human Services have compiled a guide to daily food choices, the food pyramid. The food pyramid delineates the major food groups—fats, bread, vegetables, fruit, milk, and meat—as well as the number of recommended daily servings. Each section of the pyramid is a food group. The size of the section indicates the number of recommended daily servings. The smaller the section, the less you should eat of that type of food. At the broad bottom of the pyramid is the bread group, which should comprise a large part of your diet. On the other hand, notice that fats, oils, and sweets occupy a small section at the top. This means you should use fats and sweets sparingly.

The food pyramid. (Source: U.S. Department of Agriculture and the U.S. Department of Health and Human Services)

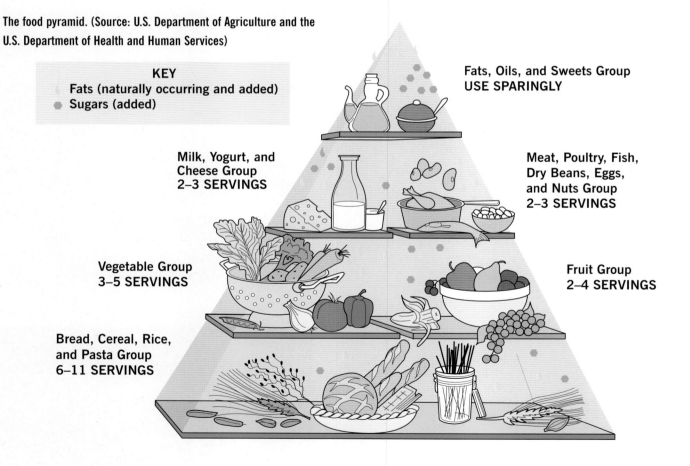

KEY
Fats (naturally occurring and added)
Sugars (added)

Fats, Oils, and Sweets Group
USE SPARINGLY

Milk, Yogurt, and Cheese Group
2–3 SERVINGS

Meat, Poultry, Fish, Dry Beans, Eggs, and Nuts Group
2–3 SERVINGS

Vegetable Group
3–5 SERVINGS

Fruit Group
2–4 SERVINGS

Bread, Cereal, Rice, and Pasta Group
6–11 SERVINGS

What nutrients does each food group provide?

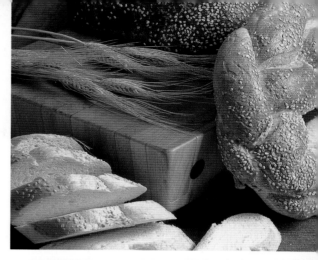

BREAD GROUP (6–11 servings/day). Provides complex carbohydrates, fiber, and vitamin B.

Serving size: 1 slice of bread; ½ plain bagel; muffin or bun, 1 cup ready-to-eat cereal; ½ cup rice; pasta; or cooked cereal.

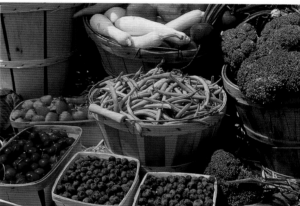

FRUIT GROUP (2–4 servings/day). Provides vitamins A and C, folate, potassium, and fiber.

Serving size: 1 cup raw, leafy green vegetables; ½ cup other vegetables, cooked or raw, including potatoes.

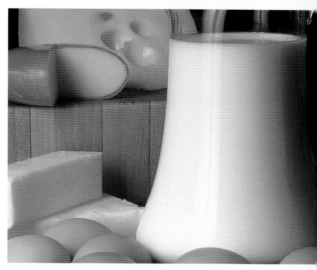

MILK GROUP (2–3 servings/day). Provides protein, calcium, and vitamins A and D.

Serving size: 1 cup milk or yogurt; 1–2 ounces of cheese; and ½ cup cottage cheese.

MEAT GROUP (2–3 servings/day). Provides B vitamins, protein, iron, and zinc.

Serving size: 3 ounces cooked and boneless lean red meat; skinless poultry or fish; ½ cup cooked beans; 1 egg.

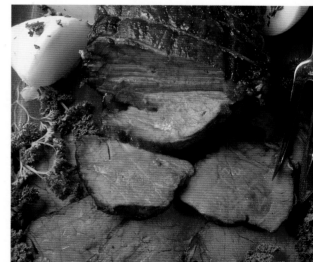

FATS, OILS, AND SWEETS (0–1 servings/day). Eat less foods like oil, salad dressing, or butter. Soft drinks, candies, and cookies are high in sugar. Eat less of this group.

Serving size: 1 teaspoon.

Food choices

What is a serving size? A serving is generally 3 ounces. This is roughly what you can cup in the palm of your hand.

Please refer to Appendix C for vitamin and mineral sources, as well as examples of easy-to- prepare nutritious meals. Most importantly, avoid foods that are fried or are served with cream sauces or butter, as well as high-Calorie snacks and desserts.

If you like to eat out, simply substitute low-fat items for high-fat items. For example:

Choose	Instead of	To save
1 Tbsp. low-fat cottage cheese	1 Tbsp. butter	67 Calories and 9 grams of fat
½ cup cereal with 1 percent low-fat milk	½ cup cereal with whole milk	24 Calories and 3 grams of fat
1 Tbsp. low-fat salad dressing	1 Tbsp. regular salad dressing	66 Calories and 7 grams of fat
3-oz. chicken thigh, no skin, roasted	3-oz. chicken thigh, with skin, fried	57 Calories and 5 grams of fat

Eating Sensibly

A sensible diet program, which includes energy proportions for performance, includes 60 percent from carbohydrates, 15 percent from proteins, and no more than 25 percent from fat. An easy way to improve your knowledge of food Calories, fat grams, and nutrients is to read the food labels on packaged food.

If your goal, for example, is to have no more than 25 percent of your Calories come from fat on any given day, and your total energy intake is 2,000 Calories, then 500 Calories of fat, or 55 grams of fat, is the daily amount you need.

2,000 Calories x 0.25 = 500 Calories of fat per day

500 Calories of fat per day ÷ 9 (Calories ÷ grams of fat)
= 55 grams of fat per day

Sports activities differ widely in the amount of energy (food Calories) required to support them. In general, sports require a greater caloric intake than the sedentary life. Carbohydrate-rich foods can increase glycogen, a stored energy source in muscles, for the athletic individual. Foods high in fat leave the stomach slowly and may contribute to a persistent feeling of fullness.

Nutrition Facts

Serving Size ½ cup (114g)
Servings Per Container 4

Amount Per Serving

Calories 260   Calories from fat 120

	% Daily Value*
Total Fat 13g	**20%**
Saturated Fat 5g	25%
Cholesterol 30mg	**10%**
Sodium 660mg	**28%**
Total Carbohydrate 31g	**11%**
Dietary Fiber 0g	0%
Sugars 5g	
Protein 5g	

Vitamin A 4%	Vitamin C 2%
Calcium 15%	Iron 4%

*Percent Daily Values are based on a 2000 calorie diet. Your daily values may be higher or lower depending on your calorie needs.

	Calories:	2000	2500
Total Fat	Less than	65g	80g
Sat. Fat	Less than	20g	25g
Cholesterol	Less than	300mg	300mg
Sodium	Less than	2400mg	2400mg
Total Carbohydrate		300g	375g
Dietary Fiber		25g	30g

Calories per gram:
Fat 9 • Carbohydrate 4 • Protein 4

Exercising then may be unpleasant. Protein is a major structured component of all body tissue and is needed for growth and repair. Interestingly, proteins are inefficient sources of energy and are used for energy only when sufficient sources of carbohydrates and fat are not available. Compare the typical diet with the high-activity diet:

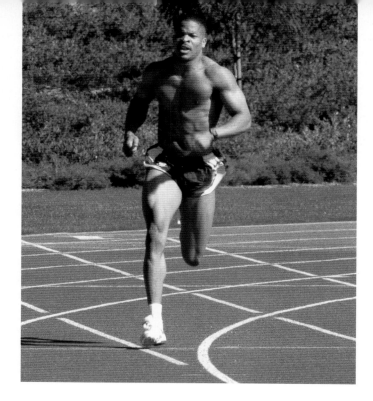

Food component	Typical diet (percentage of total daily Calories)	Suggested diet for high activity (percentage of total daily Calories)
Protein	10–15	15
Fat	30–40	20–25
Carbohydrates	45–50	60–65

Note: To convert grams to Calories, multiply grams of protein x 4.3, grams of fat x 9.3, and grams of carbohydrate x 4.1.

Summary

The most successful way to maintain your weight, lose weight, or gain weight is very simple:

➤ Keep a food diary and monitor your food intake.

➤ Exercise at a moderate level of intensity most days of the week.

➤ Have a good support system such as family and friends to help keep you on track.

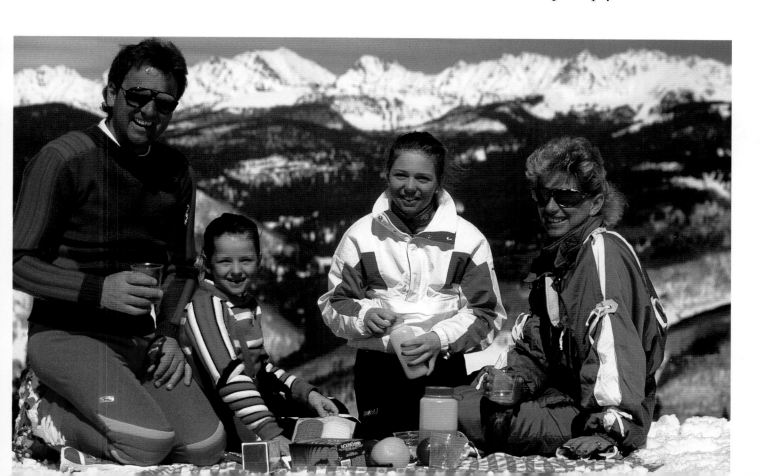

The Mind

The brain requires more oxygen than any other organ of the body because of its high rate of metabolism. A common remedy for stress is to breathe deep, supplying the brain with increased oxygen and thereby improving mental balance, concentration, and emotional control. In addition, deep breathing improves the physical control and coordination needed in most sports.

Breathing

Proper breathing primarily involves the movement of the diaphragm muscle. During inhalation, the diaphragm descends and the abdomen expands, drawing air in through the nose and filling the airways within the lungs. As air moves into the alveoli in the countless number of small air sacs inside the lungs, oxygen from the air is transferred to the blood. During exhalation, as the diaphragm rises, old air filled with carbon dioxide is pushed out of the lungs with the help of the intercostal muscles.

Along with daily exercise and a balanced diet, proper breathing helps us to achieve a sense of enhanced well-being and increased energy. In addition, relaxation is very helpful in clearing the mind and allowing us to become the best we can be in terms of mental and physical health.

A tip for relaxation

Silence is golden. A large amount of our mental and physical energy is used up in

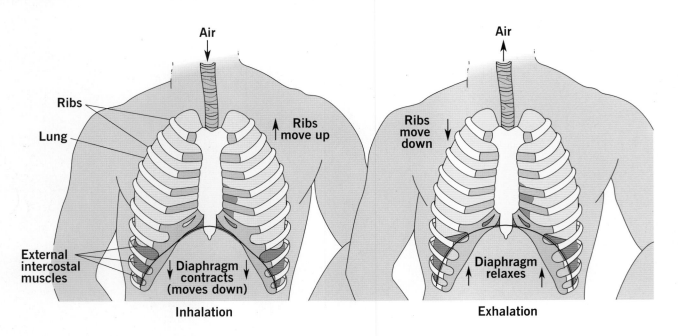

Inhalation — Air; Ribs; Lung; Ribs move up; External intercostal muscles; Diaphragm contracts (moves down)

Exhalation — Air; Ribs move down; Diaphragm relaxes

body

everyday talking and socializing. By quieting the mind, there is no better way to soothe and recharge the mind, body, and soul than by taking a few minutes each day to sit in silence. Find a quiet place to relax, a place that warms your heart and soothes your soul, and listen to inspirational music, read, watch nature, or meditate. Allow this time to be effortless. Simply marvel in the present moment, and enjoy.

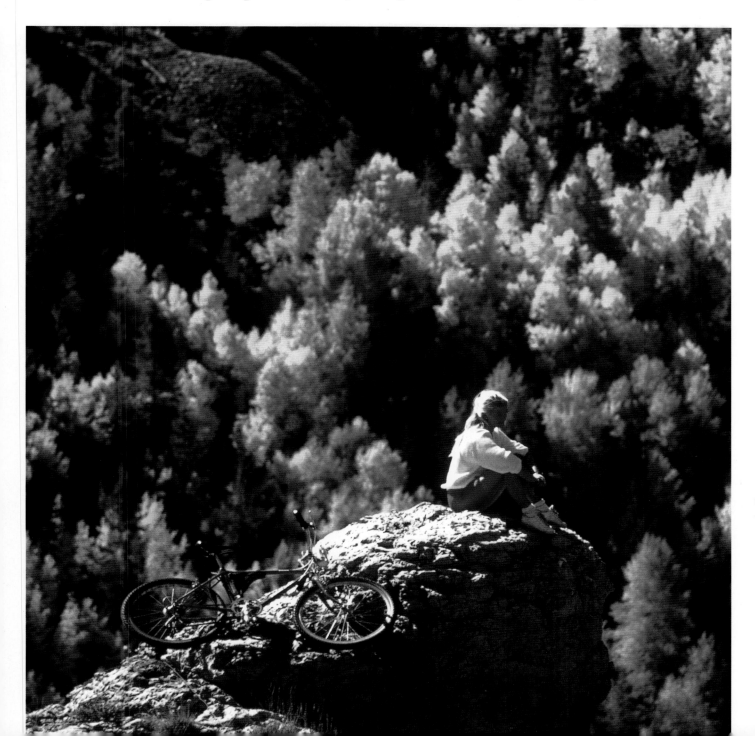

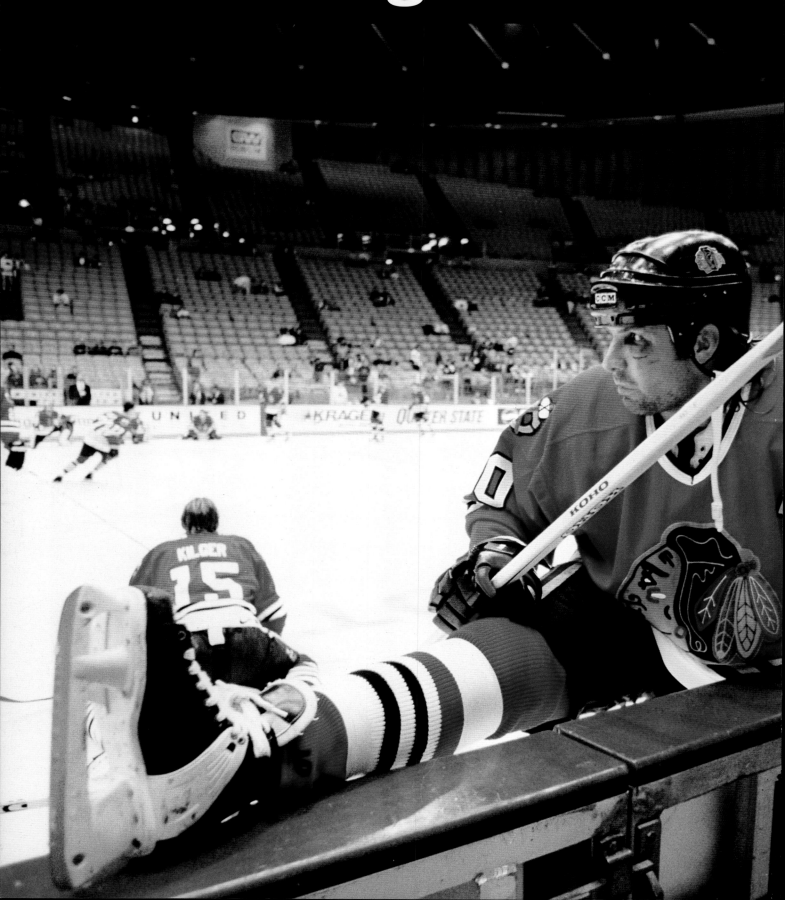

gthening

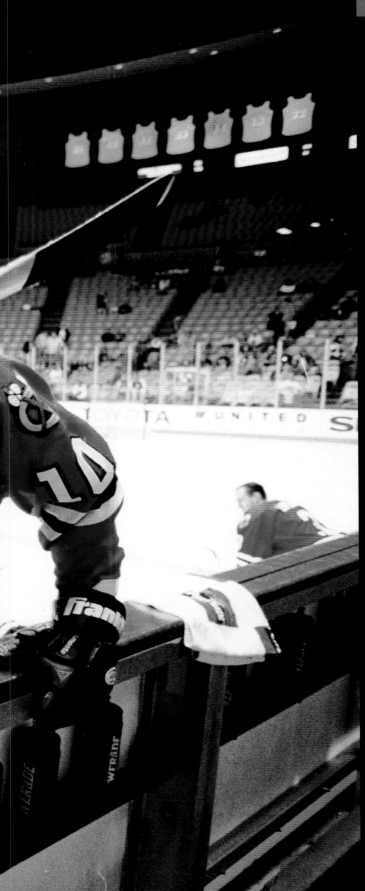

Stretching

    Upper body

    Back and hips

    Upper legs

    Lower legs and feet

Strengthening

    Back and shoulders

    Arms

    Abdominals

    Hips and legs

    Legs

    Combinations

Stretching

This part contains two sections: first, a series of basic stretches, and second, strengthening exercises, which together will prepare your muscles for any physical activity. You will improve your muscles by stretching the ones you have strengthened and strengthening the ones you have stretched. With time you will see an increase in your flexibility and power.

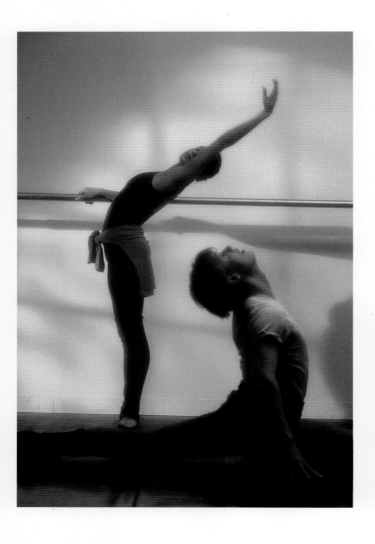

STRETCHING FOR FLEXIBILITY

Flexibility is desirable because it decreases the accumulated tension in your muscles, enables you to move more easily, and helps prevent injuries when exercising or playing sports. Flexibility is often measured in terms of range of motion. The more flexible you are, the farther and more comfortably you can move the respective joints and extend your muscles. The best way to increase flexibility is to do stretching exercises daily. Stretching also promotes good circulation and helps develop body awareness. Besides that, it just feels good.

Set aside 10 to 15 minutes every day for your routine. You may use the following stretching exercises in sequence, or use the stretch that works the body part you want to focus on. Remember to always begin your stretch after a 3- to 5-minute warm-up such as a walk or a slow jog in place.

Note: If you have been inactive or live a sedentary lifestyle, or if you have had a recent or persistent physical problem, especially of the muscles or joints, please consult your physician before starting a stretching or strengthening program.

How to stretch

As you begin to stretch, keep breathing naturally. A slow rhythmic pattern is best. Do not hold your breath while stretching. Ideally, spend 10 to 30 seconds holding a stretch, and never bounce.

Stretch to a point where you feel mild tension in the muscle. The feeling of tension should subside as you hold the position. If not, ease off on the stretch and find a level of tension that is comfortable for you. Since we all have different levels of flexibility, do not compare yourself with others. Your stretch should feel mild, without pain.

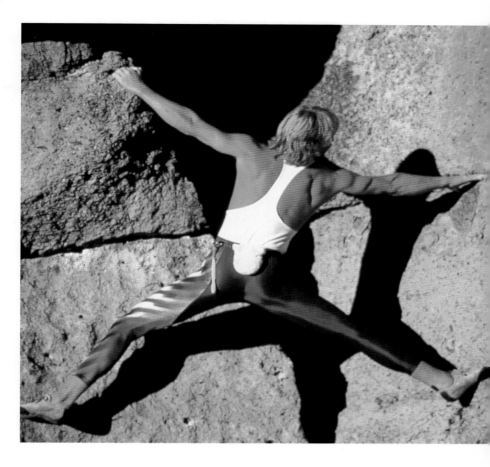

Overall body stretch

By starting your day with an overall body stretch, you will feel looser and more at ease. A good stretch will feel invigorating to tight and stiff muscles. (Hint: It may be helpful to take a hot shower to get warm before you stretch.)

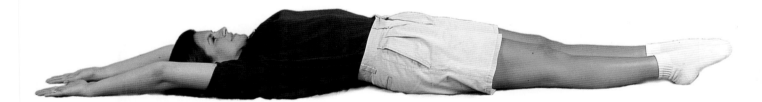

• Lie on your back, extend your arms overhead, pull in your abdominal muscles, straighten your legs, and point your toes while pushing your lower back to the floor. For 10 to 30 seconds, reach upward with your arms and downward with your toes as far as you can. Relax and repeat.

Repeat the entire stretch as many times as you like. Usually 2 to 3 times is adequate to reduce tension. This stretches the shoulders, arms, hands, feet, ankles, and abdominal muscles in addition to the rib cage and internal organs.

Upper body

Neck stretches

Perform neck stretches with caution, especially if you have any neck problems. Consult your physician if you have any questions.

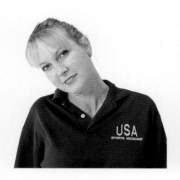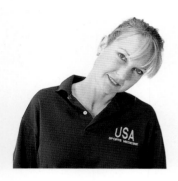

• To begin, relax the left arm and shoulder, and slowly tilt your head toward your right shoulder. Hold for 10 to 30 seconds. Repeat on the opposite side. Repeat 1 to 3 times.

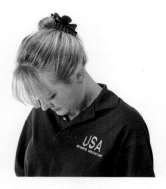

• Stand or sit with arms relaxed at your sides. Gently tilt your head forward, stretching your chin toward your chest. Feel the pull on the back of your neck. Hold for 10 to 30 seconds. Do not bounce. Repeat 1 to 3 times.

Shoulder and upper back stretches

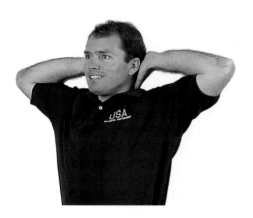

• You may do this stretch sitting in a chair or standing. Interlace your fingers behind your head. Keeping your elbows straight and out to the side, pull your shoulder blades together. Hold for 10 to 30 seconds. Relax and repeat 1 to 3 times.

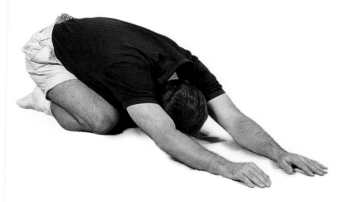

• Kneeling down, with your rear end resting on your heels, stretch your arms out in front of you. Press your upper body toward the floor. Reach your arms as far forward as you can while keeping your head down and rear end resting on your heels. Keep pressing toward the floor for 15 seconds. Sit up and relax. Repeat 1 to 3 times.

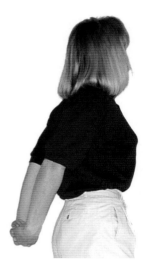

Chest and upper back stretch

• Stand with your fingers interlaced behind your back. Lift your arms up behind you until you feel a slight tension in your chest, upper back, and arms. Hold that position 10 to 30 seconds, relax, and repeat 1 to 3 times.

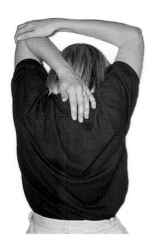

Triceps and shoulder stretch

• Raise your arms overhead and hold your left elbow with your right hand. Gently pull the left elbow behind your head until you feel a bit of tension. Do this slowly. Hold the stretch for 10 to 30 seconds, relax, and repeat on the opposite side. Repeat on each side 1 to 3 times.

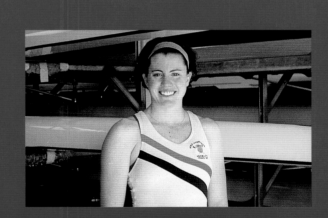

Sally Scovel, Rowing

Sally rowed competitively throughout her college career in California. In 1998, after graduation, she captured a silver medal in the World Championships in Germany and another at the World Cup in Switzerland. She went on to compete in England at the first Women's Invitational held since 1828, and she hopes to row in the 2000 Olympics.

Because her lower body gets worked so hard during training (especially her legs), she concentrates on developing her upper body strength by lifting weights and using the bench. She also spends 30 minutes a day stretching her shoulders, upper arms, upper back, and chest. No matter what your level of exercise, Sally recommends stretching before and after you work out to avoid injury. Sally also regularly works out with her teammates for fun and motivation and suggests that others might likewise benefit from working out with a friend or joining a running group or a gym.

Back and hips

Lower back stretch

• Lie flat on your back, keeping your knees bent and feet flat on the floor. Push your lower back to the floor, hold for 10 to 30 seconds, relax, and repeat.

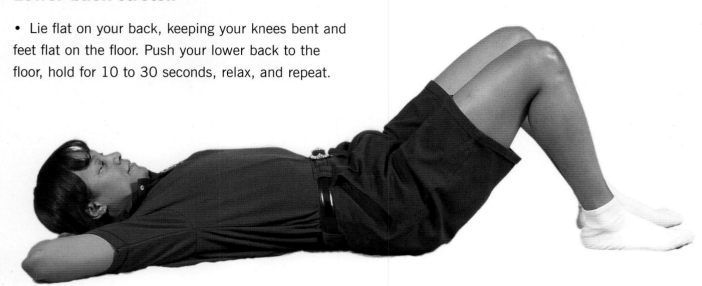

• Or you may lie down on your back, again with both knees bent and feet flat on the floor. Lift one leg and pull the knee to your chest. Press your lower back to the floor. Hold for 10 to 30 seconds. Relax. Repeat with the other leg, and relax. Repeat the stretch with both legs 1 to 3 times.

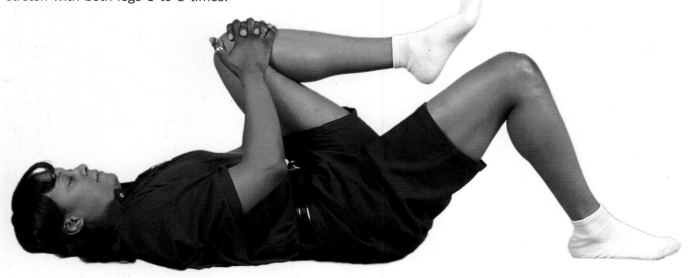

Hip and back stretch

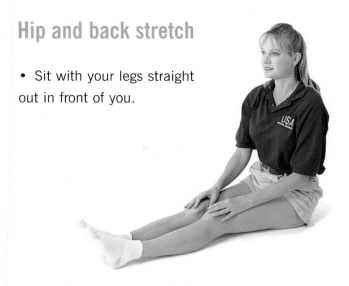

• Sit with your legs straight out in front of you.

• Bend your right knee and cross your right foot over your left leg with your right foot outside your left knee.

• Reach over and place your left elbow on the outside of the right knee. Place your right hand behind you on the floor and turn your upper body so you look over your right shoulder. Hold for 10 seconds.

Relax, then repeat on the opposite side. Repeat the entire stretch 1 to 3 times.

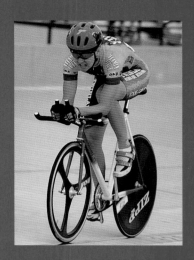

Karen Dunne, Cycling

Karen Dunne is a two-time collegiate national champion and an all-American in cycling. As a member of the U.S. National Cycling Team, she won a bronze medal in the 1998 World Cup. Her goal is to qualify for the 2000 Olympic team.

Karen has worked hard to get fit and be injury free, but she hasn't stopped there. Her focus has changed to maintaining that fitness. She says, "My lower back has given me problems ever since I first started cycling, so I've been through a back stabilization program. I can ride pain free through consecutive training days. However, when I neglect the stretching and lower back exercises, not only do I experience back pain but also knee and/or ankle pain. The musculoskeletal structural weaknesses I have require me to maintain a rehab program in order to meet the physical demands of cycling and progress toward my goal of making the World and Olympic teams."

Upper legs

Hamstring stretch

• While sitting with your legs outstretched in a V, place the bottom of one foot against the inner thigh of the opposite, extended leg.

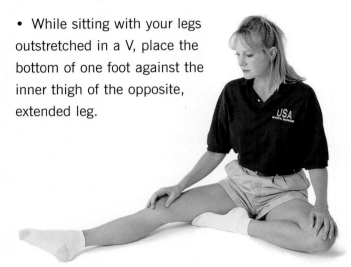

• Slowly bend forward at the hips, reaching toward the foot of your straight leg. Your arms should be outstretched and your head bent toward the knee. Hold the stretch for 10 to 30 seconds, then relax. Repeat on the opposite side. Repeat 1 to 3 times.

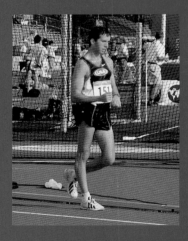

Tim Seaman, Race Walking

Tim Seaman is a member of the U.S. National Track and Field Team. He began race walking at 17 years of age and competed throughout his college career at the University of Wisconsin-Parkside, from which he graduated in 1995. Tim hopes to race in the 2000 Olympic Games; he takes inspiration from the 1996 Olympic gold medal race walker Jefferson Perez.

Tim's approach: "Always put stretching into your training program, start your program off slow, and if you do feel pain, stop, rest, and use the RICE principles (see page 76)." In his routine, Tim stretches the groin, hips, and legs along with the other major muscle groups before and after each exercise session. One of his favorite stretching exercises is the hamstring stretch. In 1998 he had pelvic surgery to correct a tendon and muscle injury, which he attributes in part to overtraining and tight muscles.

Quadriceps stretches

• Stand on your left leg with your left hand at your side or resting on a nonmoving support. Bend your right knee and grasp your right foot with your right hand. Gently pull the foot upward and hold it for 10 to 30 seconds. Relax, then repeat on the opposite side. Repeat the stretch on both legs.

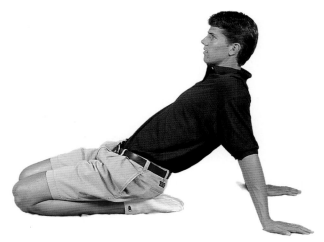

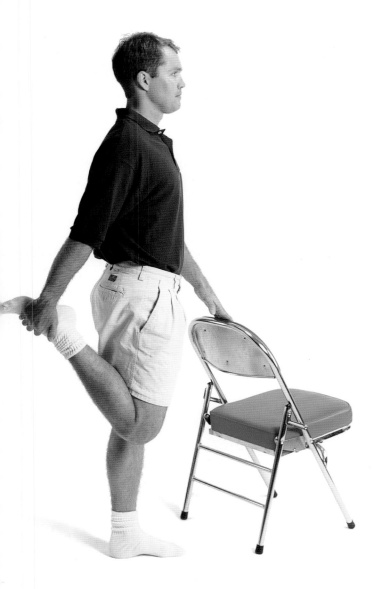

• Alternatively, while sitting with your rear end resting on your heels, place both arms behind you on the floor and extend your arms backwards until you feel tension in your quadriceps. Hold the stretch for 10 to 30 seconds, then sit up and relax. Repeat 1 to 3 times.

Hip and inner groin stretch

• Sit on the floor. Place the soles of your feet together, and draw your feet toward you as close as is comfortable. Keep your back straight. Place your hands on your knees and gently press down. Hold for 10 to 30 seconds. Relax, and repeat 1 to 3 times.

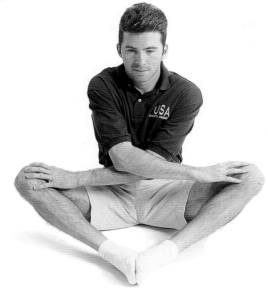

Lower legs and feet

Standing calf stretch

• Stand away from a wall or stable support and lean on it with your forearms. Place your left foot in front of you, with the leg bent. Hold your right leg straight behind you.

Slowly move your hips forward until you feel tension or stretching in the lower calf. Hold this stretch for 10 to 30 seconds, and then relax. Repeat, using the opposite leg. Remember not to bounce. Repeat the stretch 1 to 3 times on each leg.

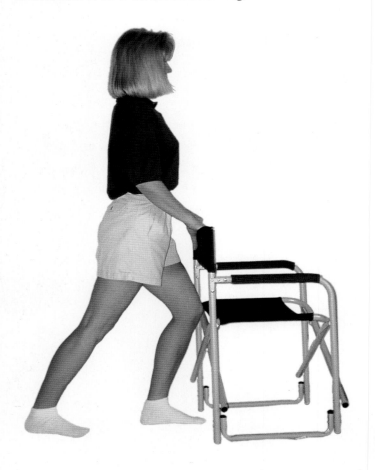

Calf and Achilles tendon stretch

• Stand with your feet slightly apart. Lower your hips and slide your right leg straight behind you while supporting your trunk and upper body over the opposite bent knee. Keep both heels flat on the ground. The Achilles tendon only needs a mild stretch. Hold the stretch for 10 to 30 seconds, then relax. Repeat 1 to 3 times on each leg.

Sitting calf stretch

• For a more advanced stretch, sit on the floor with your legs together and extended in front of you. Grab your toes and gently pull them toward you. Find a level of tension that feels sustainable, hold for 10 to 30 seconds, and relax. Repeat 1 to 3 times. To increase the stretching effect, you can lean forward at the waist.

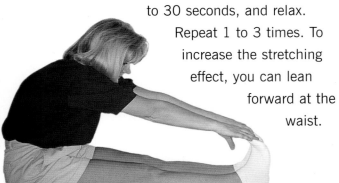

Ankle and foot stretch

• While sitting on the floor with both legs extended, bend one leg and place the ankle on the thigh of the outstretched leg. Use your fingers to pull the toes of your bent leg toward you to stretch the top of the foot and the tendons of the toes. Hold for 10 to 30 seconds, relax, and repeat. Then rotate your ankle clockwise and counterclockwise through a complete range of motion. Repeat the stretch on the opposite side. Repeat the entire stretch 1 to 3 times.

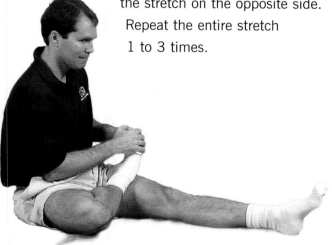

Foot arch stretch

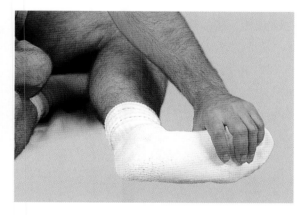

• Using your thumb or fingertips, massage up and down the longitudinal arch of your foot. Use circular movements with a good amount of pressure to loosen the ligaments. Do both feet about 30 seconds to 1 minute.

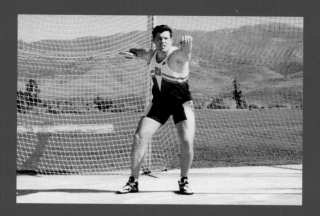

Kevin Fitzpatrick, Discus

Kevin Fitzpatrick placed third in the 1994 U.S. Olympic Festival, second in the 1995 U.S. Olympic Festival, and seventh in the 1996 Olympic Trials. He is a current hopeful for the 2000 Olympic Games.

Kevin began throwing for fun as a young child, but he threw rocks, much to his parents' concern. When his brother and his father came across a discus for sale at an auction, they bought it for Kevin, and his career was launched. While in college at the University of Tennessee, Kevin participated in track and field. He loves the camaraderie of competing with the best in his field, and his desire to always do better keeps him motivated.

Kevin trains all year long and focuses, naturally, on strengthening the back, shoulders, and arms for throwing the discus. He varies the intensity of his workouts by cross training in such activities as biking, tennis, and racquetball. Kevin warms up and stretches all major muscle groups before exercise, and then cools down and stretches afterward as well. In 1998, during an explosive 200-foot throw, he experienced a partially torn calf muscle, which required surgery and extensive rehabilitation. Today he spends extra time stretching these calf muscles to avoid another injury.

Strengthening

STRENGTHENING EXERCISES

Increased muscular strength will give you more resistance to injury, and it will improve your appearance because your muscles will have tone. You'll also have more energy, endurance, and strength to participate in sports and a variety of other physical activities. In short, you'll feel and look better.

For most sports and for general fitness, a strength-training program should include at least one exercise for each major muscle group. You can perform exercises with or without equipment to develop muscular strength. Always seek advice from a professional sports trainer if you have questions or if you are just starting out.

There are three basic types of strengthening exercises: isometric, isotonic, and isokinetic. *Isometric exercises* involve creating

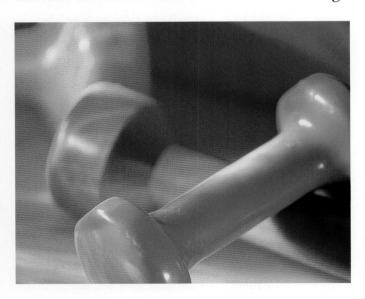

tension in muscles by pushing against a stationary object such as a wall, a door frame, or a nonexercising limb, contracting the muscle but not moving the joint. They are very useful for maintaining muscle tone without the use of equipment and may moderately improve muscle strength. In contrast, *isotonic exercises* involve active movement such as lifting free weights or doing push-ups. The muscles contract during the exercises. *Isokinetic exercises* involve constant resistance through a full range of motion, using sophisticated and expensive equipment generally not available to the recreational athlete. This section provides isometric and isotonic strengthening exercises suitable for most sports.

Before lifting weights, learn and follow the proper techniques to prevent injury. If you choose to lift weights, start with only enough weight that is comfortable for you, then advance to more weight as you become stronger. The last repetition of a set of strengthening exercises should feel difficult to do, but as you make progress it will feel easier, and you will be ready to increase the weight. Remember to stretch 15 to 20 minutes before and after your strengthening program. When lifting weights, always inhale at the start of the lift, and exhale as you finish. Do not hold your breath. Never twist or suddenly jerk when lifting weights. These movements could cause a muscular injury.

Strengthening program

A good strengthening program follows the "FIT" guidelines discussed in Part II (see page 30). FIT is an acronym that stands for Frequency, Intensity, and Time, three factors in training for fitness or athletic performance that you can vary to suit your personal objectives.

In terms of frequency, you should schedule your strength-training workout three times a week, with one day of rest between your workouts. A 24-hour rest period allows your muscles to adapt to training and build new tissue. Strength gains are achieved by the intensity of your workout. Not everyone should train at the same intensity. As a general guideline, the amount of weight you lift should be between 50 and 80 percent of the maximum weight you can comfortably lift. You should add weight gradually, and only when you are ready. For example, if you can perform twelve repetitions three times in several workouts, you should be ready to add more weight to your strengthening program. Time does not play as important a role in building strength as frequency and intensity. You should feel *no* pain on your

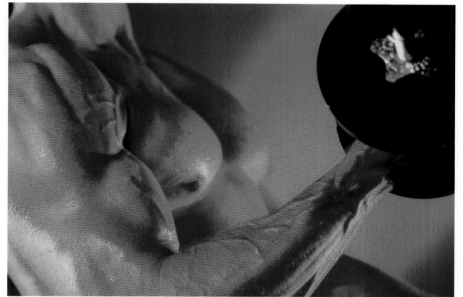

rest day—perhaps only a little discomfort and a sense of body awareness. If you feel stiff or sore, cut back on the intensity of your program.

Dangers of anabolic steroids

Unfortunately, the use of anabolic steroids is on the rise, in part because of the popularity of body building. It must be emphasized that the use of anabolic steroids has serious health consequences, and there is no need to depend on steroids—or any drug—for strength or performance.

The harmful effects of steroids on the body include high blood pressure and heart disease; liver damage; male reproductive diseases such as decreased sperm production, testicle shrinkage, and testicle and prostrate tumors; female masculinization, including increased body hair, menstrual changes, and voice deepening; psychological changes and mood swings; inability to fight infections; and the weakening of tendons and ligaments.

The International Olympic Committee and the United States Olympic Committee ban the use of anabolic steroids by Olympic athletes or any other athlete.

Back and shoulders

Strengthening the back and shoulders

➤ REVERSE FLY

• Lie face down on a bench, grasping a 3-pound dumbbell in each hand. Begin with your arms hanging straight down (not shown). First bend your arms, then slowly raise them out to each side, parallel to your chest, contracting the shoulder blades. Hold that position for 3 seconds, then lower your arms to their starting position, and repeat 8 to 12 times.

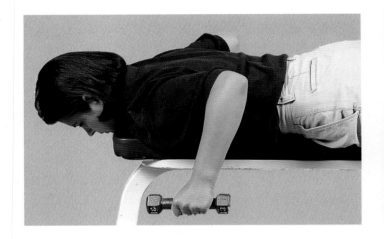

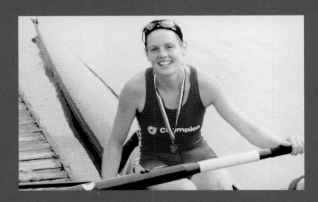

Michelle Borkhuis, Rowing

Michelle Borkhuis participated in rowing throughout her college career at the University of Massachusetts. After graduation in 1996, she won a gold medal in the Canadian Henley Games, and in 1997 she was a three-time gold medalist in lightweight women's eights at the Nationals and a silver medalist in women's lightweight pairs at the World Championships. In 1998 she won a bronze medal in the lightweight class at the Worlds and a silver medal in open women's pairs at the Nationals.

Michelle naturally focuses on building upper body strength, but an essential part of her training program is stretching the back and shoulders before and after exercise, which for her is key to preventing recurring injury. She keeps motivated to train by clearly outlining her goals and working toward them. In addition to her training as a rower, Michelle keeps fit all year round by running and biking.

Strengthening the arms and chest

➤ KNEE PUSH-UPS

• Beginners usually start by doing knee push-ups. Get down on your hands and knees, with the hands parallel to each other and no more than shoulder width apart. Lower your body until your chest touches down. It should only brush the floor. Then push yourself back up to the starting position. Repeat 8 to 12 times.

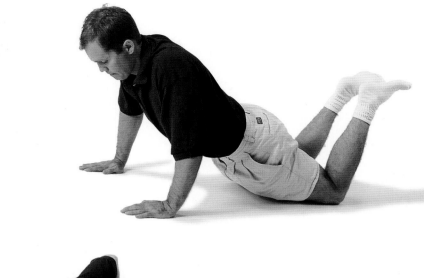

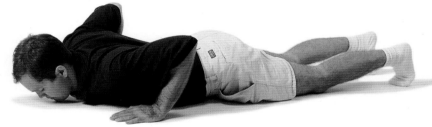

➤ FULL PUSH-UPS

• When you feel strong enough, try a full push-up. Place your legs straight behind you with your back straight and your head up. As you inhale, lower yourself until your chest touches the floor. Pause, then exhale while pushing back up to the starting position. Repeat 8 to 12 times.

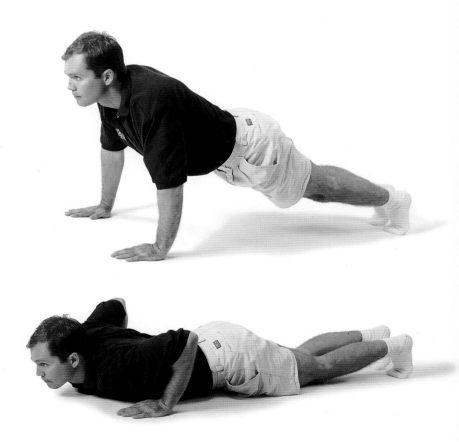

Arms

Strengthening the biceps

➤ BICEPS CURLS

• Start out using light
weights, such as a
1-pound to 3-pound
hand weight or
dumbbell. Stand
with your knees
slightly bent. Hold
the dumbbells in
front of your thighs
with an underhand grip.

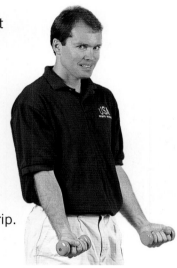

• Slowly curl both arms
up to chest level. Hold
for 3 seconds, then
lower. Repeat for 8
to 12 repetitions.
Remember to
breathe: Inhale
as you raise the
dumbbells and
exhale as you
lower them.

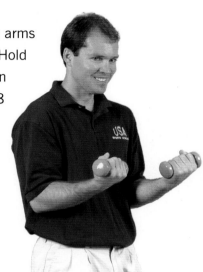

Strengthening the biceps and forearms

➤ FRENCH CURLS

• Stand upright, with your
abdominal muscles tight.
Holding a 1-pound to
3-pound dumbbell in
each hand with an
underhand grip, keep
your elbows close to
but not touching
your body. Allow
your forearms to
hang loosely
away from your hips.

• Without moving your
upper arms, curl the
weights diagonally into
your chest until the
knuckles of each hand
face each other.
Slowly lower the
weights to your starting
position. Repeat 8 to
12 times.

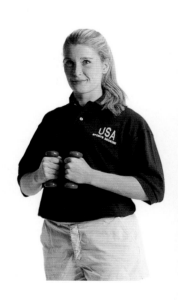

Strengthening the triceps

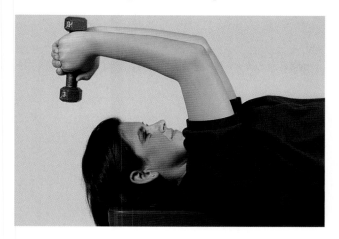

> O V E R H E A D   E X T E N S I O N S

• Start out using a pair of 3-pound to 8-pound dumbbells. Lie face up on a bench. Raise both arms perpendicular to your chest and hold one dumbbell in each hand. With the upper arm stationary, lower your forearms until they are parallel to the bench. Continue lowering the dumbbells as far as you can without moving your upper arms. Hold for 3 to 5 seconds before raising your arms to the starting position. Repeat 8 to 12 times.

Strengthening the fingers, hands, wrists, and forearms

> R U B B E R   B A L L   S Q U E E Z E

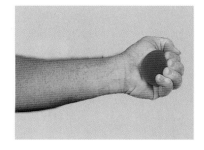

• By using a 2½-inch-diameter rubber ball, you can strengthen your fingers, hands, wrists, and forearms. Squeeze the ball in one hand, using all your fingers and the thumb, until you tire. Relax and repeat 6 to 12 times. Switch to the opposite hand and repeat 6 to 12 times.

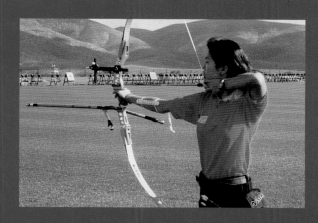

Jo-Ann Malahy, Archery

Jo-Ann Malahy is a three-time all-American and a two-time collegiate national champion (1997) in indoor and outdoor archery. In 1998 she was one of three American women elite archers to obtain a score of 1300 out of 1440 possible points (the world record is 1378 points). During the last two years she has competed at the international level, and she hopes to bend her bow for the U.S.A. in the 2000 Olympic Games.

Jo-Ann considers archery an endurance sport. In training, she may stand in one position for as long as six hours a day. She says that she needs strong back muscles to prevent injury and her faith to give her spiritual strength and guidance. She concentrates on stretching and strengthening her back and shoulders, although she also stretches all major muscle groups before and after she exercises. To keep fit, she cross trains by race walking, biking, and running. Because archery requires a focused mind, Jo-Ann practices daily mental imagery and visualization exercises.

Abdominals

Strengthening the abdominal muscles

➤ HALF SIT-UP

• Lie on your back with knees bent and feet flat on the floor and pulled toward the buttocks, hands across your chest.

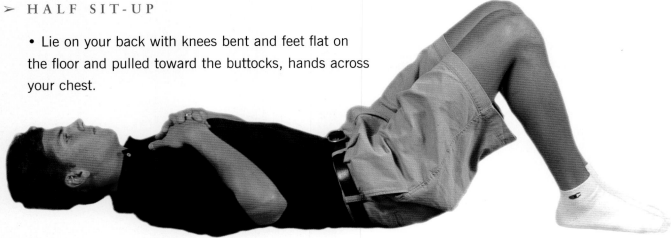

• Keeping your head in a fixed position, lift your head and the top of your shoulders off the floor. Keep your chin tucked as you lift your shoulders. Hold this position for 5 seconds, then return to your starting position. Repeat 6 to 12 times.

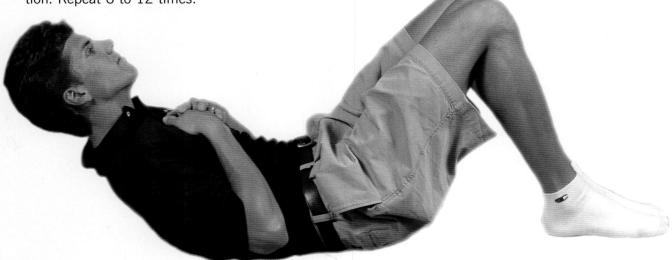

ALTERNATING ELBOW/KNEE ABDOMINAL CURLS

• Lying on your back, interlace your fingers behind your head. Raise your feet off the floor, bend your knees, and raise them vertically above your hips. Bring your upper body to about a 30-degree angle from the floor.

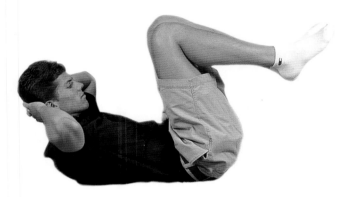

• Touch your right elbow to your left knee, then touch your left elbow to your right knee. This is one count. Do 3 to 6 repetitions. This alternating abdominal curl takes more strength and coordination than simple abdominal curls.

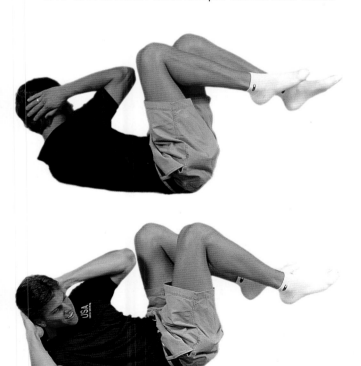

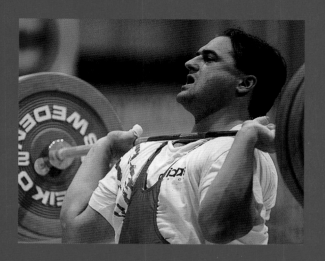

Pete Kelly, Weight Lifting

Pete Kelly started lifting weights at the age of 13 with the dream of playing football. As he began getting stronger, he increased the weight he was lifting, and he was soon asked to join the school weight lifting team. During his high school career, Pete won a variety of Junior National competitions, and by his junior year he was competing in the 90-kilogram weight class.

After graduation, he was accepted at the Colorado Springs Olympic Training Center to continue training for national and Olympic contests. In 1996 Pete broke five national records and was a contender in the 1996 Olympics in the 99-kilogram weight class.

Pete presses as much as 400 pounds. He understands that, although his spinal column and back muscles have to be strong to support that kind of weight, having strong abdominal muscles is important to stabilize the back. Pete works his abdominals hard on a daily basis, doing sit-ups and other strengthening exercises. Before working out, however, Pete always stretches all major muscle groups.

Pete's advice: Just push yourself to work up to your limit; don't overdo it. Keep a regular schedule and results will follow.

Hips and legs

Strengthening the hip extensor and gluteals

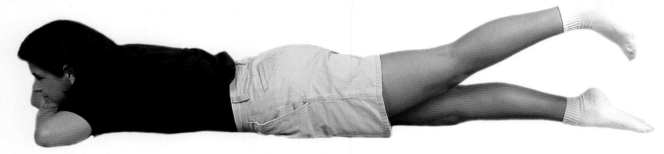

➤ LYING HIP RAISE

• Lie face down with your chin resting on your hands. With the hips pressed to the floor, slowly raise one leg 2 to 4 inches, keeping the leg straight. Don't arch your lower back. Hold that position for 2 seconds and then lower the leg. Do the exercise with your other leg and repeat, alternating legs with each repetition. Repeat 6 to 12 times.

Strengthening the quadriceps

➤ CHAIR LEG RAISES

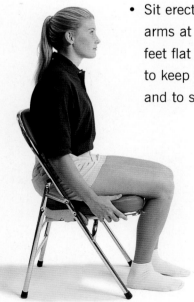

• Sit erect in the chair, with your arms at your sides and your feet flat on the floor. Remember to keep your hips stationary and to sit evenly.

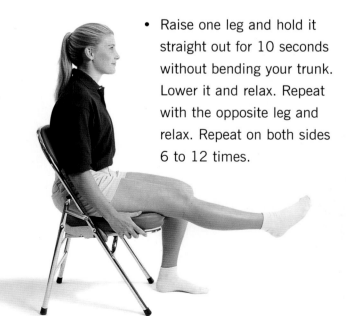

• Raise one leg and hold it straight out for 10 seconds without bending your trunk. Lower it and relax. Repeat with the opposite leg and relax. Repeat on both sides 6 to 12 times.

Strengthening the hip abductor and outer thigh

➤ LEG LIFTS

• Lie on your right side with the right leg bent at a 45-degree angle and your body weight supported by your left arm as shown.

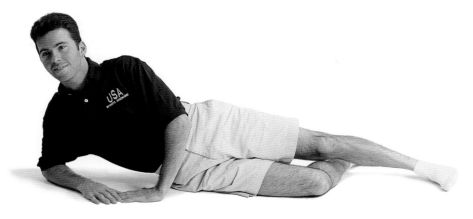

• Keeping the left leg straight, raise it to hip level or higher if you can. Hold the leg raised for 20 seconds. Relax and repeat 6 to 12 times. Switch to the opposite side and repeat 6 to 12 times.

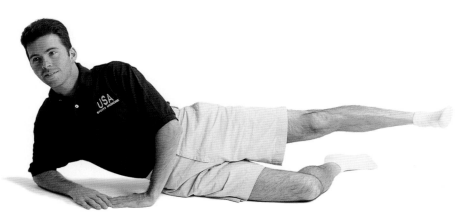

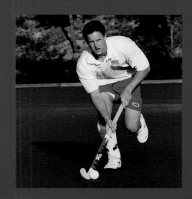

Steve Danielson, Field Hockey

Steve Danielson has been playing field hockey since he was 10 years old. A member of the 1996 U.S. Olympic Field Hockey Team, he hopes to qualify for the 2000 Olympic team as well.

Steve advises everyone to stretch a minimum of 15 minutes before exercise (he himself likes to stretch 30 minutes or more before and especially after exercise) to prevent injury. In early 1998, Steve had arthroscopic surgery to repair an injury to his right hip and then participated in six weeks of rehabilitation. Since the injury, Steve has concentrated even more on stretching his hips and legs than he did before. Steve also cross trains by running in the pool and using a stationary bike all year round. To stay confident and focused in his sport, Steve regularly participates in mental imagery and visualization exercises.

Legs

Strengthening the inner thigh

➤ LEG RAISE

• Lie on your right side and bring your left knee in front of your right hip.

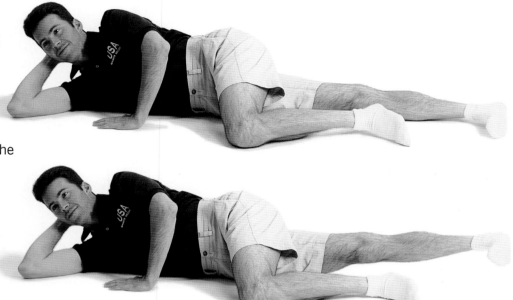

• With the foot flexed and the toes pointed, raise your left leg as shown, and hold that position for 5 seconds. Relax, then repeat 6 to 12 times. Relax again, then switch sides, repeating the exercise 6 to 12 times.

Strengthening the lower leg

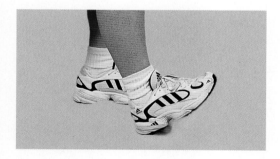

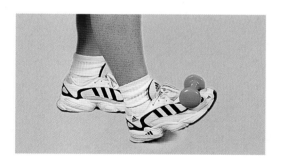

➤ TOE LIFTS

• With the heel of one foot on the ground, gently raise the toes toward your shin and let them down again. Do this 20 times. Switch feet and repeat.

• You can also do toe lifts with weights, although no more than 3 to 5 pounds is recommended. Using a dumbbell to increase the intensity of this move helps balance the stronger calf muscles in the back of the leg and strengthens the front lower leg muscles, which helps prevent painful shin injuries.

Combinations

Strengthening the arms and legs and improving coordination

> COMBINATION ARM
> AND LEG LIFT

By using a large inflatable Swedish ball, you can increase strength while improving your overall coordination and stability. In this exercise, it is recommended that you work with a partner to stabilize your position at all times.

Note: Contact your local athletic store to purchase a specifically designed, strong Swedish ball (inflatable). A simple beach ball is not strong enough to support weight.

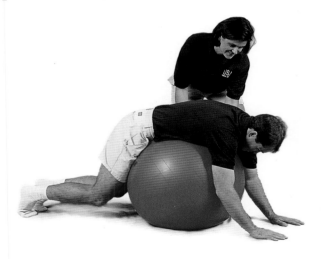

• Kneel over the ball with your midsection resting on the ball. Your hands and feet should be resting comfortably on the floor.

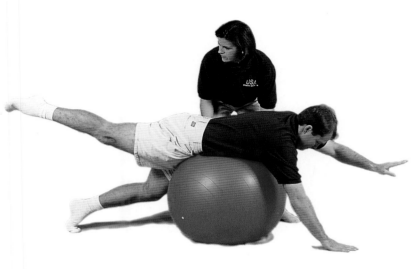

• Simultaneously raise your right leg and left arm while squeezing your gluteal muscles (buttocks) as your leg lifts. Hold for 15 seconds. Relax and return to the starting position, then repeat, using your left leg and right arm. Do the entire exercise 6 to 12 times.

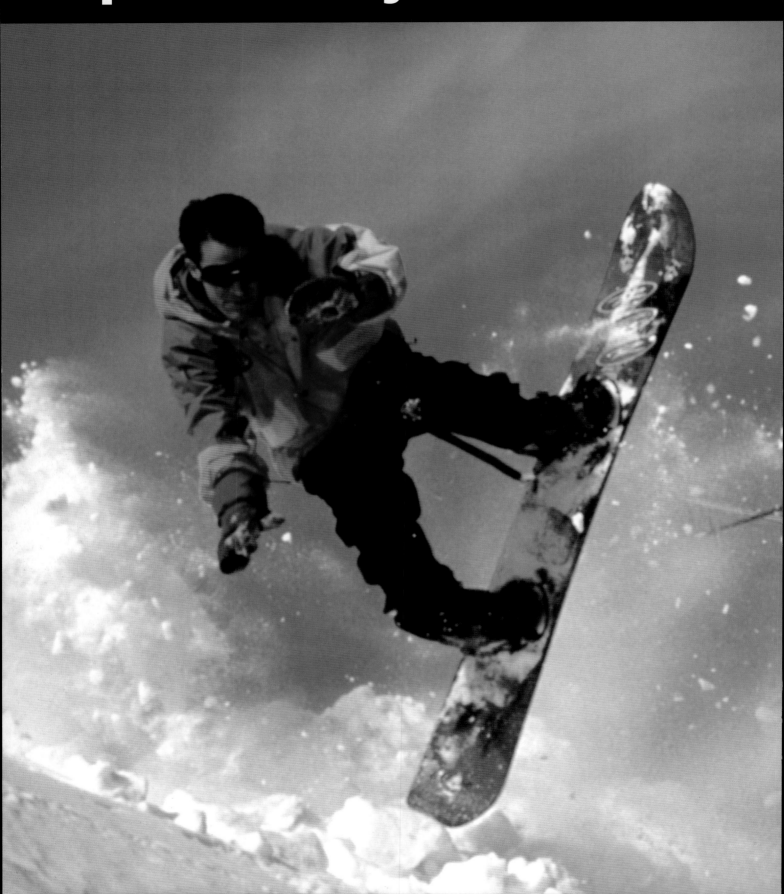

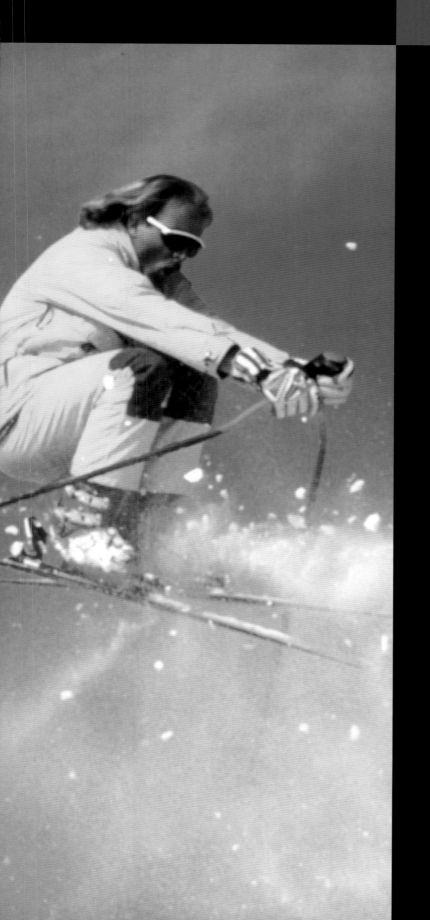

Understanding injury

Prevention, care, and rehabilitation

Head and neck

Shoulders, upper back,
   and chest

Upper extremities

Abdomen

Lower back and hips

Thigh

Knee

Lower leg, ankle, and foot

Understanding injury

Whether you're an Olympian training for an international competition or a working adult trying to get in a handful of 30-minute workouts each week, your motivation is to be fit and healthy. You don't want injuries. The more insight and understanding you have about sports injuries, the more active a role you can play in preventing them, treating them if they do occur, and getting rehabilitated so you can play again or return to your full workout. More specifically, by understanding the cause of a sports injury the better prepared you will be to prevent the injury from recurring.

There are three basic causes of sports injury. All of them can occur alone or in combination.

1. Stress or overuse of a body part is the most common cause. Any cumulative, repetitive motion that causes tissue damage can lead to overuse injuries. Throwing a softball and taking an overhead swing in tennis are examples of

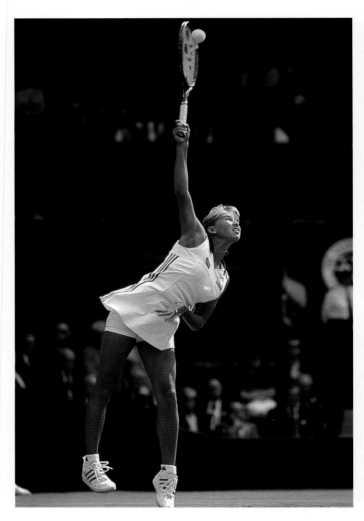

Repetitive motion such as overhead swings in tennis can cause overuse injuries.

DISCLAIMER: Neither Part IV, Sports Injuries, nor any other part of this book is intended to substitute for medical consultation or the recommendation of a physician. Since the field of exercise and injury care is continually changing, the reader should always consult with his or her physician, sports trainer, or other health professionals before starting any nutrition, exercise, or injury-care program.

such repetitive motion. Chronic overuse from these activities can create an imbalance between groups of muscles that rotate the shoulder, leading to inflammation of the connective tendons, called rotator cuff tendinitis. Other examples of sports-related repetitive motion injuries are runner's knee, shin splints, and tennis elbow.

2. Coordination failure when you make a sudden twist or drastic movement is another leading cause of sports injury. For example, during a basketball game, if a player leaves his lower legs planted while he rotates his upper body, this can create undue stress across the knee ligament, resulting in a torn ligament (sprain), a fracture (broken bone), a dislocation, or a combination of all three.

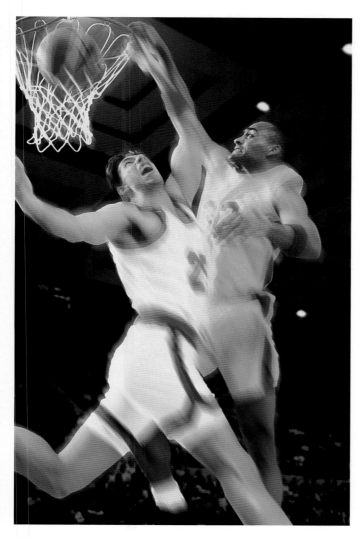

Sudden twists or drastic movements stress joint ligaments.

3. Direct trauma—a sudden collision with another object—is the third common cause of sports injury. Obviously, this happens frequently in contact sports like ice hockey and football. In football, this type of injury could be caused by blocking or tackling another player, by your body hitting the ground, or by collision with another player.

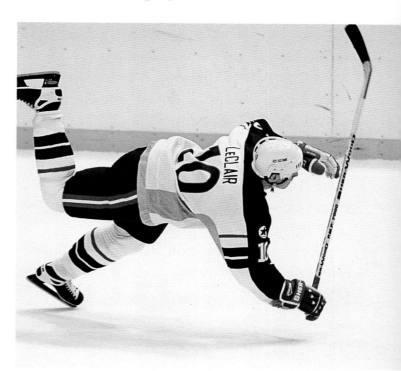

Falls or collisions produce direct trauma.

Defining a sports injury

Injuries can be categorized as soft tissue injuries or skeletal injuries. Both kinds of injuries can occur suddenly, as in an acute injury such as a broken bone, or over time, as in a chronic injury caused by overuse. Runner's knee is a good example of continuous repetitive movement wearing out part of the body a little at a time.

SOFT TISSUE INJURY What is soft tissue? The body's soft tissue consists of muscles, tendons, ligaments, nerves, blood vessels, fat, fascia, and skin. Internal body organs such as the liver, spleen, stomach, and intestines are also soft tissue but will not be discussed.

Muscles make up approximately 30 percent to 40 percent of an adult's body weight. Voluntary muscles called skeletal muscles are connected to the various bones by tendons. Blood vessels and nerves are woven between the muscle fibers. Muscle fibers that make up a muscle work by either shortening (contracting) or lengthening (relaxing). Impulses from a nerve cause the muscle to contract. The fascia, which is a strong, fibrous tissue, gives support and holds soft tissue, nerves, and blood vessels together.

Strong ligaments hold the bony skeletal joints together, as demonstrated by the knee joint ligaments. Ligaments keep joints stable and mobile.

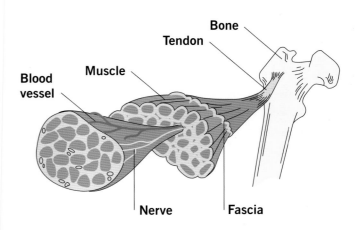

A skeletal muscle attaches to the bone by a tendon and other soft tissues—the fascia, blood vessels, nerves, and muscle fibers.

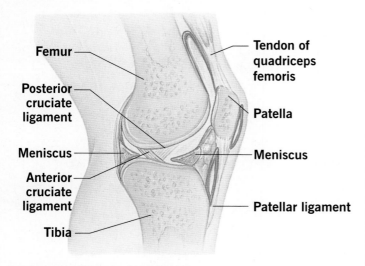

Strong knee ligaments keep the joint stable and mobile.
From *Human Anatomy & Physiology*, by Elaine Marieb; copyright © 1989, Benjamin/Cummings Publishing Company, Inc. Reprinted by permission.

HUMAN SKELETON The human skeleton with its 206 bones (this number can vary slightly from person to person) helps shape, support, and protect body structures. Bones and muscles interact to allow the body coordinated movement. The bones and muscles function as levers to move the body. In addition, long bones contain tissue that produces the body's blood cells and various salts.

Rating injury severity

Prompt recognition and proper diagnosis and treatment are necessary for adequate healing and quick recovery from a sports injury. The Injury Severity Guidelines are a quick reference for classifying an injury and getting proper medical attention. These guidelines are not intended as a diagnosis. Always seek professional medical advice for moderate to severe injuries.

Injury Severity Guidelines

Injury severity	What to do

Mild
Mild pain only after exercise
Activity not affected
No tenderness to touch
No swelling
No skin color changes
No deformity

← RICE (page 76)
Medication (page 76)
Reduce activity
Return to activity slowly

Moderate
Pain before and after exercise
Activity affected
Area tender to touch
Mild swelling
Mild change in skin color
No deformity

← RICE (page 76)
Medication (page 76)
No activity
Gradual return to modified activity;
    when ready, return to full activity
Modify exercise to reduce recurrent stress
Seek medical advice

Severe
Pain before, during, and after exercise
Activity affected
Normal daily activity affected by pain
Severe pain to touch
Swelling
Skin discoloration
Deformity

← Stop activity
See doctor immediately

A Medical Emergency
Any alteration in consciousness
Drowsiness, disorientation
Seizures, altered vision
Breathing difficulties (always considered an
    emergency after injury to the head, neck, or chest)
Clear fluid draining from nose or ears
Bleeding with or without deep wound
Severe pain
Blunt injury to abdomen is considered a medical
    emergency until cleared by a physician

← Call for immediate medical attention
Do not move individual until trained
    medical professional gives the okay

CARING FOR INJURIES

What you can do for a mild to moderate injury

The most common method for treating a sports injury is RICE. RICE stands for Rest, Ice, Compression, and Elevation, shorthand for the steps you should begin as soon as an injury occurs and continue through the first 24 to 48 hours after the injury. Sometimes the acronym PRICE is used instead. The difference is that P stands for Protect from further harm and R stands for Restrict further activity. However, in this book we use RICE throughout. The most important function of RICE is that it controls and decreases inflammation and swelling, leading to a faster recovery. Remember that this is not a substitute for professional medical care.

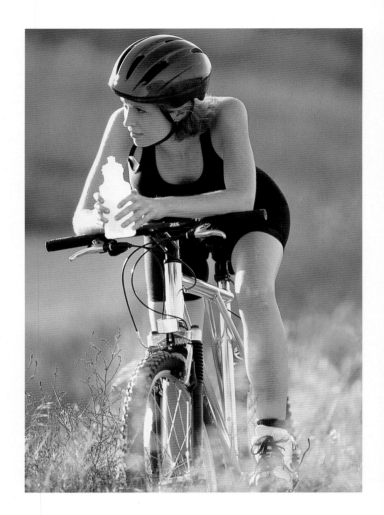

Rest	Stay off your injured ankle, foot, or leg. Rest your extremity, upper or lower.
Ice	Apply ice. (Place ice in a plastic bag or wrap it in a towel, place a wet cloth over the injured area, then the ice bag. Leave the ice on for 20 minutes, then take it off for 40 minutes. Repeat.) Icing is helpful during the first 24 to 48 hours after an injury. Some experts suggest that icing may be beneficial for up to seven days, depending on the injury.
Compression	Lightly wrap the injured area with a compression bandage.
Elevation	Elevate the injured area. Keep the upper extremities raised above the heart, and the lower extremities above the waist. This will help reduce swelling and pain.

Over-the-counter medication

On occasion, medication is required to help ease the pain and swelling of an injured area, even when using the RICE principles. If needed, and only under the direction of a physician, an antiinflammatory oral medication can be used.

Several of the over-the-counter anti-inflammatory products contain the active ingredient ibuprofen. Check with your doctor before using any of these medications because they are not risk free. They should be avoided all together if you have stomach problems or allergies to aspirin or if you are pregnant.

A tablet or liquid containing the active ingredient acetaminophen is sometimes recommended for pain control. Acetaminophen does not control inflammation and is not recommended if you are pregnant or nursing, except under a physician's guidance.

Prevention

Prevention is the most effective way to deal with exercise problems. By following a few basic guidelines, you should be able to stay injury free. If you are just beginning an exercise program, an easy way to avoid problems is to plan for gradual progress. Too little may be better than too much. After several weeks your body will feel stronger, and you will be able to increase your exercise intensity.

Modify your physical activity if you experience a sports injury. If you play a sport, consult with a sports specialist or coach to check your technique, or if you work out, to help you perfect your routine. This will help avoid repeated injury.

Whether you are a semiprofessional athlete or a weekend warrior, the following guidelines will help you avoid injury and enjoy overall continual success and health in your sport or activity.

1. Start your workout with a warm-up that includes stretches (see Part III, pages 46–69).

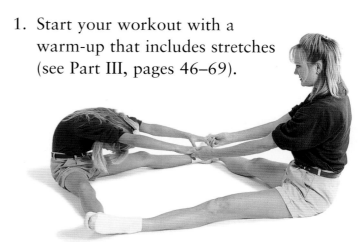

2. Avoid sudden or dramatic changes in your workout, such as running on new terrain or quickly increasing the mileage of your run.

3. Build enough rest into your workout schedule.

4. Drink plenty of water.

5. Wear the proper shoes and clothing.

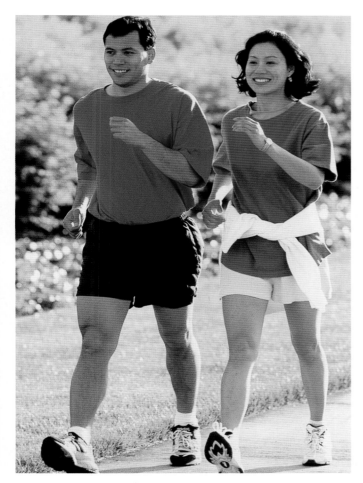

By following a few basic guidelines, you can enjoy an exercise program free from injuries.

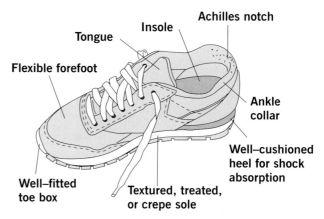

Characteristics of a proper walking shoe.

6. Maintain good flexibility.

77

SOFT TISSUE INJURIES

The body's soft tissue is made up of ligaments, tendons, muscles, nerves, blood vessels, fat, fascia, and skin. A variety of injuries can occur to these tissues when exercising or playing a sport. The Common Soft Tissue Injuries chart (see pages 80–81) lists some of the most common soft tissue injuries and provides recommendations for care according to the severity of the injury (also see the Injury Severity Guidelines). It will serve as a concise and easy reference when you want to check out injuries to specific body areas.

The human muscular system

The human body has three types of muscle tissue: skeletal muscle, cardiac muscle, and smooth muscle. The three types of muscle tissue differ in their structure, location, and function. Cardiac muscle is found only in the heart, and smooth muscle is found in

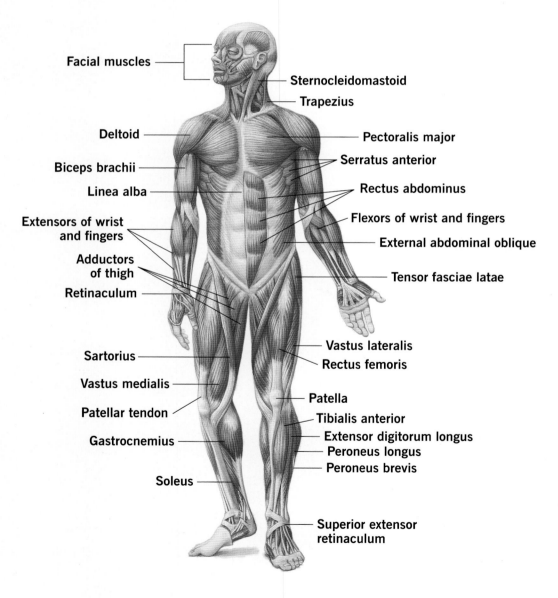

Facial muscles

Sternocleidomastoid

Trapezius

Deltoid

Pectoralis major

Serratus anterior

Biceps brachii

Rectus abdominus

Linea alba

Flexors of wrist and fingers

Extensors of wrist and fingers

External abdominal oblique

Adductors of thigh

Tensor fasciae latae

Retinaculum

Sartorius

Vastus lateralis

Rectus femoris

Vastus medialis

Patella

Patellar tendon

Tibialis anterior

Gastrocnemius

Extensor digitorum longus

Peroneus longus

Peroneus brevis

Soleus

Superior extensor retinaculum

The human superficial muscular system, front view.

the walls of internal organs such as the stomach, intestines, and urinary bladder. The cardiac and smooth muscles are not under our conscious control and are called involuntary. The skeletal muscles are attached to and cover the bony skeleton, and they give the body its mobility. These muscles are under our conscious control and are called voluntary.

In regard to sports injuries, we discuss the skeletal muscles only. Because there are more than 600 human skeletal muscles, we can't review them all, but the major skeletal muscles are covered in the descriptions of sports injuries and their care and rehabilitation. For reference, and to show how groups of muscles interact, the accompanying illustrations present the superficial skeletal muscles of the front and back of the body (deeper skeletal muscles lie underneath). Detailed illustrations of the structure and function of the various body areas accompany the respective discussions of injuries to those areas.

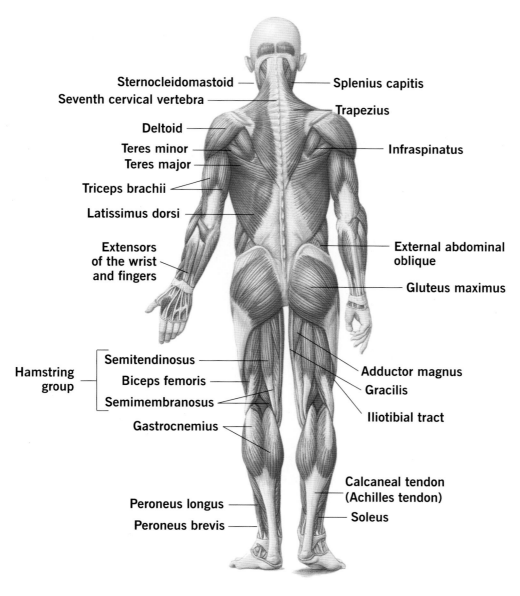

The human superficial muscular system, back view.

Common Soft Tissue Injuries

Injury	Severity level	Care
Contusion: A bruise, usually caused by a blow, in which the skin is not broken, but clotted blood accumulates under the skin.	Mild acute	Ice, rest
	Mild chronic	RICE. Seek medical attention.
	Moderate to severe (acute or chronic)	RICE. May need to seek medical attention.
Inflammation: A local reaction in blood vessels and tissue in response to injury, abnormal stimulation, or a physical, chemical, or biological agent. Area is red, swollen, and warm.	Mild acute	Ice, rest
	Mild chronic	RICE. Seek medical attention.
	Moderate to severe (acute or chronic)	RICE, oral antiinflammatories. Seek medical attention.
Hematoma: A localized mass of blood, usually due to a blow, that is partially or completely confined within a tissue space or organ. Forms a solid swollen area, with pain and limited motion.	Mild acute	RICE. Never use massage in the first 48 to 72 hours.
	Mild chronic	RICE. Seek medical attention.
	Moderate to severe (acute or chronic)	RICE. Seek medical attention.
Bursitis: Inflammation of the bursa, caused by friction. The bursa is a small, fluid-filled sac that lies between a bone and a tendon.	Mild acute	Oral antiinflammatories
	Mild chronic	Oral antiinflammatories. Seek medical attention.
	Moderate to severe (acute or chronic)	This inflammation could be due to infection. Seek medical attention.
Tendinitis: Inflammation of a tendon with pain and swelling	Mild acute	RICE in first 24 to 72 hours. Correct the cause of the problem.
	Mild chronic	If no relief with above, seek medical attention.
	Moderate to severe (acute or chronic)	Seek medical attention.

Injury	Severity level	Care
Tendon strain: Overstretch or tear of a tendon. Partial rupture of a tendon is a 1st- or 2nd-degree tear. 3rd-degree tear is a complete tear.	Mild to moderate (acute or chronic) Severe	RICE. Seek medical attention. Seek immediate medical attention.
Ligament strain: Stretch or tear of a ligament. 1st- and 2nd-degree tears are partial. 3rd-degree tears are complete.*	Mild to moderate (acute or chronic) Severe	RICE. Seek medical attention. Seek immediate medical attention.
Muscle strain: Overstretch or tear of a muscle. 1st-degree micro tears of muscle tissue usually due to overuse.** 2nd- and 3rd-degree strains range from severe overstretch to complete tear.	Mild acute Mild chronic Moderate to severe (acute or chronic)	RICE during first 24 hours. Symptoms leave in a matter of days. Continue with gentle exercise. Seek immediate medical attention. May need surgical repair.
Muscle cramps: Usually due to vigorous sports that have fast stop-and-go movements like handball, football, and aerobics. May be due to failure to warm up, dehydration, or running faster than in training.	Mild to moderate (acute) Mild chronic Moderate chronic Severe	Stretch muscle gently. If it persists, consult an athletic trainer and/or physical therapist and/or physician for review.

* For further discussion of sprains, see wrist sprain (page 103) and ankle sprains (page 133).
** For further discussion of muscle strain, see common thigh injuries (page 116).
Caution: If you have questions about the symptoms or proper care of an injury, or if self-help measures fail to improve the condition within a reasonable amount of time (one to four weeks), always seek advice from your doctor and sports trainer.

Note: Acute = a sudden injury. *Chronic* = injury symptoms lasting continuously for more than one to four weeks. Refer to the Injury Severity Guidelines (page 75) to review the terminology and recognition of mild, moderate, and severe injuries as well as medical emergencies.

SKELETAL INJURIES

Fractures

A broken bone generally is classified by the cause and nature of the break. A traumatic fracture is due to injury, whereas a spontaneous, or pathologic, fracture is due to disease. Fractures are also classified as to whether the bone breaks through the skin. An open, or compound, fracture is one in which the broken bone breaks through the skin and is exposed. This type of fracture can lead to infection, since bacteria can enter through the broken skin. A closed fracture is one in which the broken bone does not break through the skin.

It is important to note that when a fracture occurs, the surrounding soft tissue (muscles, blood vessels, tendons, and so on) is also damaged. For example, in an avulsion fracture, the tendon is pulled from the bone, taking with it a piece of the bone.

IMMEDIATE MEDICAL CARE
Fractures need *immediate* medical evaluation. For the bone to heal properly, sometimes the break and surrounding area need to be properly set, or aligned.

HOW FRACTURES HEAL Fracture repair depends upon several factors. For example, bones of the upper extremities

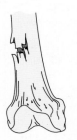

Greenstick fracture: Incomplete fracture

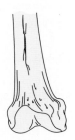

Fissured fracture: Incomplete fracture, longitudinal break

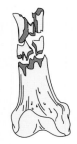

Comminuted fracture: Complete fracture with bone fragments

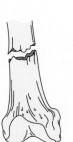

Transverse fracture: Complete fracture across bone

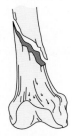

Oblique fracture: Complete fracture, occurs at oblique angle

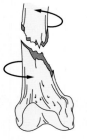

Spiral fracture: Complete fracture caused by twisting

Types of fractures.

General Healing Times for Sprains and Fractures

Type of injury	Time
*Sprain**	
1st-degree sprain (ligament stretch or tear of 25% of fibers)	5–14 days
2nd-degree sprain (half of fibers torn)	14 days–2 months
3rd-degree sprain (complete tear of ligament)	2 months–1 year
Fractures	
Wrist	10–12 weeks
Finger	3–5 weeks
Upper arm	8–12 weeks
Lower leg	12–15 weeks

Note: Healing time can vary widely, depending on the location, damage, type, and severity of the injury. Always check with your physician before returning to your regular activity or sport after any injury.

* For further discussion of sprains, see Common Soft Tissue Injuries chart (pages 80–81) and ankle sprains (page 133).

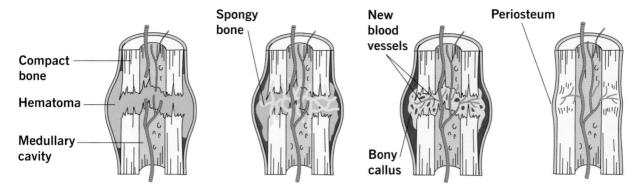

Compact bone

Hematoma

Medullary cavity

Spongy bone

New blood vessels

Periosteum

Bony callus

How fractures heal. Major steps in repair of a bone fracture.

heal in half as much time as the bones of the lower extremities. Healing is more rapid if the broken ends are close together or if a cast or metal pins are used to keep the ends of broken bones together.

The healing of a fracture is a dynamic process involving the formation, laying down, and growth of a new bone.

A dislocation requires evaluation and care by a physician to avoid reoccurrences and possibly arthritis.

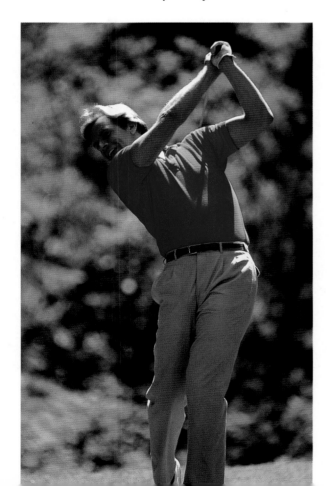

Dislocations

A dislocation occurs when a joint (two bones articulating with one another) separates. This usually means part of a ligament is torn, and surgery is required. When a dislocation is partial, meaning that there is not a full separation of the joint cavity (called subluxation), generally the joint will go back into place naturally. If these subluxations reoccur, the joint surface will wear down, leading to a condition known as arthritis. To prevent long-term wear and tear and the chronic subluxation of a joint, surgery is sometimes recommended.

Stress fractures

Stress fractures generally occur when a bone is overloaded by repetitive force (for example, by the repetitive pounding motion of running). Slight cracks in the surface of the bone occur (a plain film X ray may not be able to detect this injury), and the bone will weaken and eventually break. Risk factors for stress fracture include lack of balance, inadequate muscle stretching before exercise, wearing improperly fitting shoes that don't absorb shock, using improper

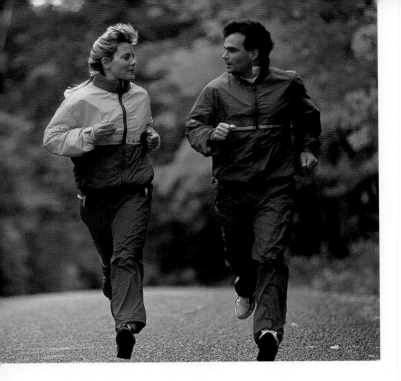

Repetitive pounding can create stress fractures.

equipment, and playing or running on an irregular surface. Always seek medical attention when you have persistent pain over the weight-bearing bone.

Other sport-related injuries

BLISTERS   A blister is a fluid-filled vesicle that forms within or under the skin in response to excessive rubbing or pressure. Foot blisters can be quite painful, and generally the culprit is improperly fitting shoes, or poor-quality socks. Never break the blister, because this can cause infection. Cover the blister with an antiseptic solution. Prevent blisters by wearing properly fitting shoes and socks, or cover the foot or hand with an adhesive pad before exercise.

LACERATIONS   A laceration is a cut to the skin, causing pain and rapid bleeding. No matter how small or where they occur, cuts need to be treated immediately to con-

trol bleeding and to prevent infection. To stop bleeding, apply pressure on the cut. Usually bleeding is controlled in 5 to 10 minutes. If bleeding does not stop, or if the cut is deep, long, or jagged, seek emergency medical attention. After bleeding has stopped, clean the cut with soap and water and cover it with a sterile bandage. You can help prevent cuts by wearing gloves, goggles, a helmet, a face mask, or whatever protective equipment is appropriate for a particular sport.

SUNBURN   Skin exposure to excess ultraviolet radiation from the sun causes inflammation of the skin. Symptoms generally are seen 1 to 3 hours after exposure and can be quite painful, depending on the depth of the

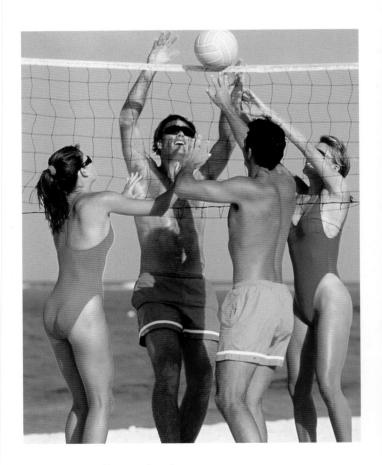

Remember to wear sunscreen.

burn. Always wear a sunscreen with a sun-protection factor (SPF) between 15 and 45. In Appendix E you will find more information on preventing sun damage and ways to recognize skin cancer.

ABRASION Abrasions are places where the surface of the skin has been scraped, exposing underlying tissue. Abrasions are very common and easy to care for. Remove any debris from the wound, and flush it with an antiseptic solution such as hydrogen peroxide. Clean the abrasion with soap and water, and cover it with an antiseptic ointment. You may cover the area with gauze. Monitor for infection. If infection develops, with increased redness and an oozing pustule, seek medical attention.

INSECT BITES Bites generally present few problems aside from itchiness and annoyance. However, some people are allergic to insect bites, and some allergies can be life-threatening. To decrease inflammation and itching, take an over-the-counter antihistamine and apply ice. If you experience any shortness of breath or swelling in the throat or face, seek medical attention as soon as possible.

HEAT-RELATED ILLNESS Exposure to high temperature characteristically produces headache, dizziness, confusion, and a slight rise in body temperature, and in severe cases, collapse and coma. If you see an athlete with these symptoms, immediately move the stricken person to a cool place, elevate the legs 8 to 12 inches, and give him or her a commercial electrolyte drink, or use cold water mixed with salt (about ¼ to 1

level teaspoon of salt in 1 quart of water). If no salt is available, give cold water. Sponge the athlete with cool water, fan him or her, and remove any excess clothing.

If there is no improvement within 30 minutes, seek medical attention. If the skin is hot, with high body temperature and altered mental status, it could signal heat stroke. Call for immediate medical attention.

INTERNAL BLEEDING This concerns bleeding within the pelvic, abdominal, or chest cavities. Internal bleeding is generally caused by a collision injury, and there are usually no external body signs. Any blunt collision injury to the body is considered *an injury needing prompt medical attention*. Signs of internal bleeding may be coughing up blood; blood in the stool; cold, clammy skin; and dizziness.

EXCESSIVE BLEEDING From a small blood capillary the blood flow will simply ooze. From a vein the blood is a dark red color and flows faster than from a capillary; and from an artery the blood is bright red and can bleed a lot, sometimes even spurting from the wound. *This is a medical emergency.* Elevate the head and keep it above the heart level. Place direct pressure on the wound.

BREATHING DIFFICULTIES Difficult breathing could be due to an allergic reaction, an exacerbation of asthma, or a heart problem. *Call for immediate medical assistance.* Keep the athlete calm and comfortable. While waiting for help, ask him or her about allergies and any medications being taken.

Prevention, care, and

This section covers the anatomy, cause, care, and rehabilitation of common sports injuries to the major body areas, including the head, neck, upper back, shoulders, chest, arms, wrists, hands, abdomen, lower back, hips, thighs, legs, ankles, and feet.

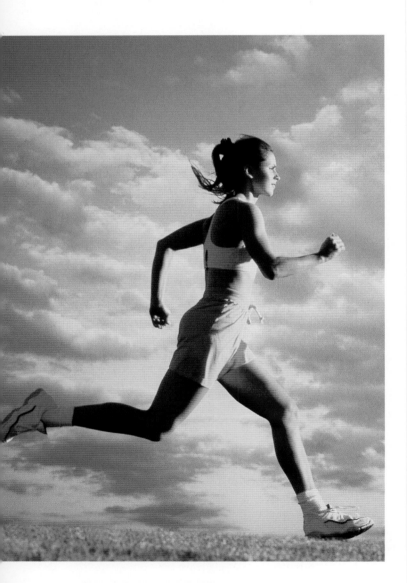

The goal of rehabilitation is to "run free" again.

Always seek professional medical advice for moderate to severe injuries. Tips on injury prevention and safety in a variety of every-day activities and sports such as running, swimming, rowing, cycling, golf, tennis, baseball, gymnastics, basketball, ice hockey, skiing, soccer, and snowboarding are featured in applications boxes. A number of Olympic athletes also offer stories of their injuries and rehabilitation and ultimate return to the Games.

Relieving the pain and symptoms of sports injury is the primary goal of injury care, but not the only one. Good care combined with rehabilitation is the "gold standard" for restoring both everyday athletes and elite athletes to their usual levels of activity. The specific goals of care and rehabilitation of a sports injury include:

1. Encouraging proper healing

2. Maintaining all-around good conditioning

3. Minimizing unwanted effects of immobilization of an injured area

4. Returning the athlete to regular activity as soon as safely possible

Today's rehabilitation programs might include techniques ranging from manual massage and manipulation to ultrasound and electrical stimulation. In the case of mild sprains and contusions, your physician may be able to recommend rehabilitation

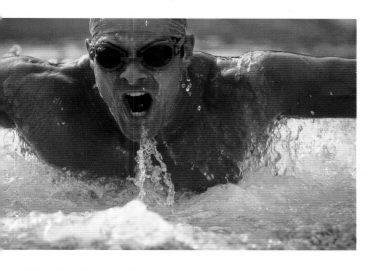

Olympic athletes offer tips on preventing injuries and recovering from them.

The time it takes you to heal is affected by factors such as your all-around physical condition, the design of your personal rehabilitation program, and your psychological well-being (see the chart of General Healing Times, page 82). Returning to your regular activities or sport should be based upon the recommendation of your physician. Usually, if 95 percent of previous function is restored to the injured site, resuming regular activities or sports is recommended.

exercises that you can do at home. If you are more seriously injured, rehabilitation is incorporated into the treatment program as early as possible in order to expedite a safe return to full activity. One of the RICE principles (the cornerstone of injury treatment) is immobilization of an injury during the first 24 to 48 hours of treatment. However, most sports doctors now recognize the benefits of early mobilization and recommend it after the initial stage of treatment to discourage loss of mobility and to promote healing. When your doctor recommends it, you may begin a rehabilitation program under the supervision of a certified athletic trainer and/or a physical therapist. They can also give you further information on specific rehabilitation methods for particular injuries.

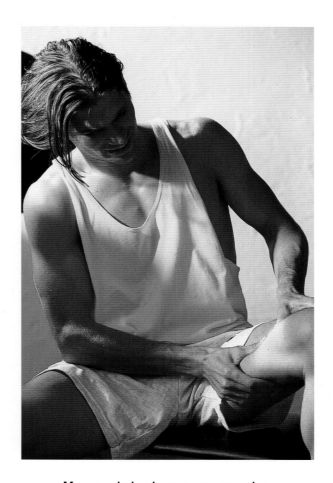

Massage helps loosen sore muscles.

Head and neck

Anatomy of the head and neck

Twenty-eight bones make up the skull (the bony portion of the head). Half of these bones are arranged into the cranial group, which contains the bones of the top, sides, and back of the head. The cranial bones primarily protect the soft tissue of the brain. The facial group of bones (fourteen in number) are the bones of your face that hold and protect the soft organs of vision, smell, and taste.

The skull is firmly attached to the topmost cervical vertebra (neck bone) of the spine called the atlas. The second cervical vertebra is called the axis. The joint between the atlas and the axis allows you to rotate your head. There are seven cervical vertebrae in all. The other five vertebrae, all with similar shapes, enable you to move your neck forward, backward, and side to side and to rotate it.

You can move your head because of the action of muscles attached to the skull and cervical spine. Unless you are lying down, these head and neck muscles are continually active keeping your head upright. Because the head needs to move in different directions and because its center of gravity is in front of the neck, the weight of your head is always pulling forward. The muscles in the back of your neck work hard to keep

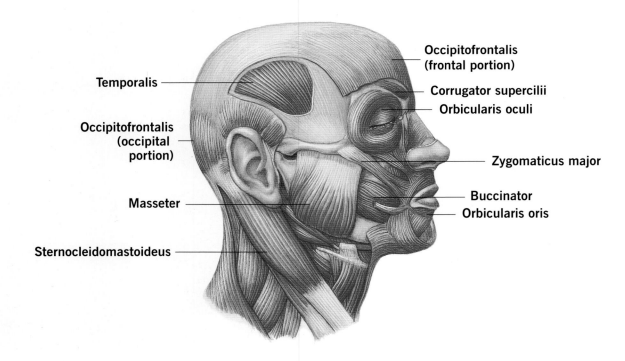

Temporalis

Occipitofrontalis (occipital portion)

Masseter

Sternocleidomastoideus

Occipitofrontalis (frontal portion)

Corrugator supercilii

Orbicularis oculi

Zygomaticus major

Buccinator

Orbicularis oris

Head and neck muscles.

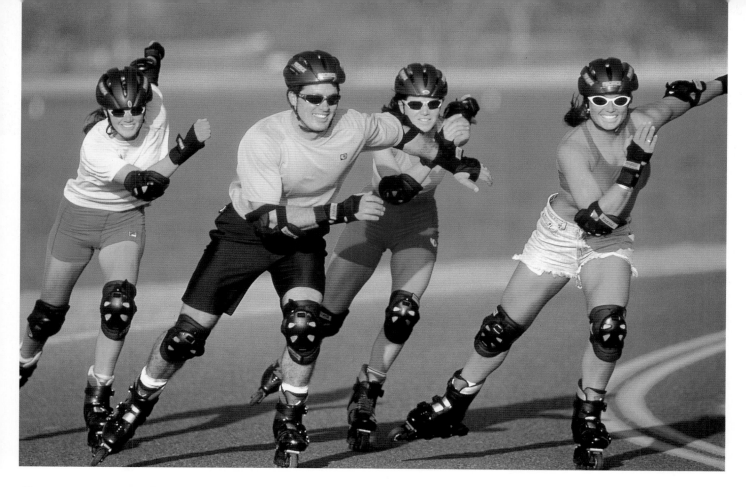

Always wear a proper-fitting helmet when roller blading, cycling, or playing a contact sport or any other sport where required by rule.

your head vertical. This is one reason why so many people suffer from tightness or soreness in the back of the neck. In fact, just sitting at a desk for prolonged periods—reviewing papers or reading a book with the head cantilevered forward—can be stressful to the neck muscles. If this happens to you, by bringing your chin in you will use the neck muscles in the front of your spine to keep your head aligned, and you should feel more comfortable.

Neck muscles differ in action. For example, forward movement is controlled by the sternocleidomastoid muscle, which is a flexor muscle, and backward movement by extensor muscles, the splenius capitis and the semispinalis capitis (see anatomy, page 109). Muscles on either side of your neck contract at the same time in opposite directions to keep the head upright.

Preventing head and neck injuries

To avoid injuries to the head or neck, understand the risk of injury in your particular activity or sport. Find out what clothing, equipment, or techniques are required and use them. For example, always wear a helmet that fits properly when cycling or playing a contact sport.

To prevent sore neck muscles, adequate stretching before and after you exercise is essential (see page 50). Neck stretches can even alleviate tension headaches caused by tight, sore muscles of the neck and head.

Common head and neck injuries

SCALP WOUNDS The scalp, which overlays the bony skull, is rich in blood supply. A blow to the head from a soccer ball, let's say, could cause a simple superficial bleeding wound without any pain or loss of consciousness. In treating these minor injuries, it is recommended to seek immediate medical attention if, upon looking into the wound, there is any tissue or skull bone exposed or if the skull has been deformed. If not, then keep the head and shoulders elevated while applying direct gentle pressure to the wound with a dry, sterile dressing. Do not remove the dressing if it becomes soaked. Add another dressing

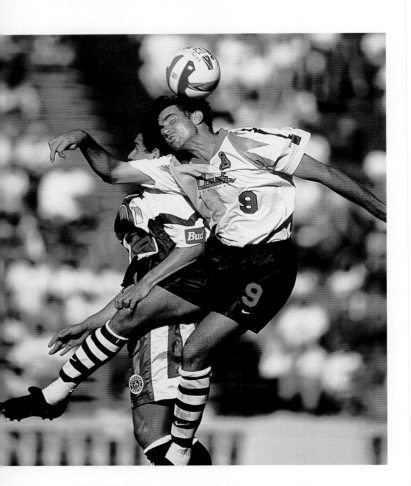

A blow to the head could cause a scalp wound.

90

on top of the first. Usually, bleeding will stop within 10 minutes. However, even if the wound is mild, seek medical advice.*

CONCUSSION A concussion comes from a severe blow to the head that results in violent jarring or shaking of the brain tissue within the skull. This may or may not cause loss of consciousness. For example, a baseball hitting your head or a sudden fall when mountain biking could cause a concussion.

If there is no bleeding or loss of consciousness and you don't suspect a spinal cord injury, then observation over the next 24 to 48 hours is advised. Use the Head Injury Follow-up Guidelines (page 92).

If any signs of concussion are present, then immediate medical care is necessary. Never move a person if there is bleeding, loss of consciousness, or a suspected spinal injury. *This would be considered a medical emergency.*

Always seek medical evaluation. Generally, in mild to moderate concussion, a physician will recommend that the injured player avoid rigorous activity for a few days or longer.

HEAD CONTUSION Contusions are more severe than concussions. Both can be produced by a blow to the head. Contusions involve bruising or swelling of the brain tissue, with blood vessels in the brain rupturing and bleeding. There is no way for the blood to escape, so it accumulates. *This is a medical emergency.* Call for immediate medical assistance. Any head injury may also be accompanied by a spinal injury, so never move the injured if you suspect this.

*When in contact with any bodily fluid, follow the universal precautions for preventing infections transmitted by blood (see Appendix I).

CYCLING SAFETY

- Always wear a helmet
- Cycle with a buddy or let someone know your travel time and route
- Always check tires for wear and cuts
- Maintain correct tire pressure
- Keep brakes adjusted
- Keep the chain, chain wheel, and rear sprocket free of dirt
- Always wear reflective clothes
- Keep flashlight handy at night
- Carry a spare tire or inner tube, a tire pump, and a water bottle

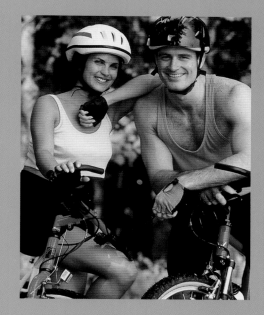

NOSE BLEED Most nose bleeds stop on their own. If a blow to the nose caused the injury, then you should seek immediate medical attention to check for a fracture. If the nose bleed persists for more than 5 to 8 minutes, seek medical attention.

For a simple nose bleed:

1. Have the injured sit down to reduce blood pressure, and keep the head tilted slightly forward.

2. Apply steady pressure to both nostrils by using the thumb and forefinger. Maintain steady pressure for at least 5 minutes. In addition to pinching the nose, applying an ice pack over the nose may help control bleeding. Remind the person to keep calm and quiet, and to breathe through his or her mouth.

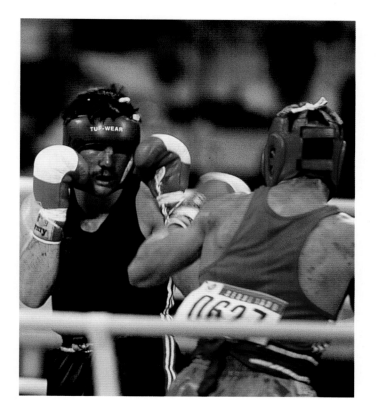

Ouch!

A person with high blood pressure or anyone taking blood-thinning medication is at particular risk for prolonged bleeding.

EYE INJURIES One of the most common injuries to the eye is an orbital hematoma, commonly known as a "black eye." This injury is generally caused by a blow to the eye, which causes pain, bruising, and swelling. Apply an ice pack for 15 minutes and seek immediate medical attention. In *all* cases of eye injury, seek medical attention, especially if there is bleeding or impaired vision.

NECK PAIN Movements that may be particularly stressful to the neck include overhead activities in sports such as tennis, swimming, volleyball, basketball, and golf.

If neck pain occurs after playing a sport and is unrelated to any trauma, the restriction of motion and pain is generally due to a muscle spasm ("wry neck"). If symptoms begin after frequent neck rotation, the neck pain could indicate a problem with the cervical vertebrae, and medical evaluation is recommended.

To relieve neck pain not associated with a blow to the neck but caused by overuse in overhead activities, rest is the cornerstone of therapy. Lying on your back in bed usually relieves local neck pain produced by muscle spasms, but it may have no effect if the bony vertebrae are involved. For tight muscles or muscle spasms, a moist warm towel can be wrapped around the neck as a collar. When the towel cools, remove it and repeat 1 or 2 times. Repeat the session every 3 to 4 hours until you feel relief. If there is no relief in 24 to 48 hours, seek medical advice.

By using proper sport technique and equipment, unwanted muscle soreness can be avoided. If a cervical spine problem is suspected, and muscle pain is not relieved by rest, seek professional medical evaluation. Always remember to wear protective equipment made spcifically for a particular sport. For example, you should always wear the right helmet for sports such as cycling, skateboarding, snowboarding, hockey, or football.

Contrary to popular belief, in-line skaters who wear a bike helmet may still be at risk for head injuries, since skaters need more protection at the back of the head than a bike helmet can provide. When selecting a helmet, choose one that meets the safety standards of the Department of

Transportation or U.S. Cycling, Inc., or seek advice from a professional sport shop.

Important: Neck injuries are often associated with head injuries because the cervical spine (the neck) supports the head. Therefore it is very important to be alert to a neck injury whenever there is a blow to the head that may involve the neck. Because the spinal cord of the neck and adjacent nerves are responsible for many vital life functions, such as breathing and heartbeat, and are also involved in thought and sensation, head and neck injuries are the most serious of all injuries.

The consequences of ignoring a neck injury can include death or permanent disability. Because of that fact, it is extremely im-portant whenever a neck injury is suspected that the injured person *not be moved.*

Fortunately, head and neck injuries are infrequent for the recreational athlete. Nevertheless, whenever there is a head injury it should be assumed that there is a high probability that it may be accompanied by a neck injury and that the injured individual has to be treated by a professional, who will assess the seriousness of the injury.

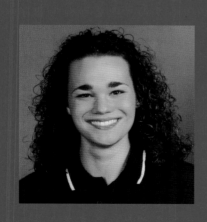

Courtney DeBolt, Volleyball

Courtney DeBolt played center on the Michigan State volleyball team. While there, she tore the anterior cruciate ligament (ACL) in both knees, which required reconstuctive surgery and extensive rehabilitation. But Courtney was determined to continue playing, and she succeeded in returning after graduation to play on a professional volleyball team in the Netherlands.

In 1996 she returned home and made the U.S. Women's National Volleyball Team. She played well but reinjured her knees in the summer of 1998, requiring a second ACL reconstruction. Each surgery and rehabilitation went well, without any major problems, although each recovery period had its "sticking points" when it was easy for her to get depressed and feel she was regressing.

Courtney says, "You need to maintain a positive attitude, trying to look at the short-range picture as well as the long-range picture, and have faith in your physician and athletic trainer or physical therapist. They will do all they can to allow you to return to your sport at the level you were prior to your injury.

Anatomy of the shoulders, upper back, and chest

The shoulder joint, more than any other joint in the body, is capable of a wide range of motion. A normal shoulder joint allows you to make a complete circle at the shoulder with your arms. Because the shoulder is so flexible, it also tends to be unstable, which can lead to a variety of problems.

The shoulder is composed of four joints, with more than 20 muscles directly or indirectly involved in shoulder action for effi-

ciency of motion. Refer to the illustration of shoulder anatomy. The shoulder bones are held together by relatively weak ligaments, which means that the ligaments are more stable if the attached muscles are kept in good condition. The muscles that surround the four shoulder joints (the glenohumeral joint, the acromioclavicular joint, the sternoclavicular joint, and the scapulothoracic joint) keep the joint stable and in position. The glenohumeral joint connects the ball of the humerus (upper arm bone) and the socket of the shoulder blade. The

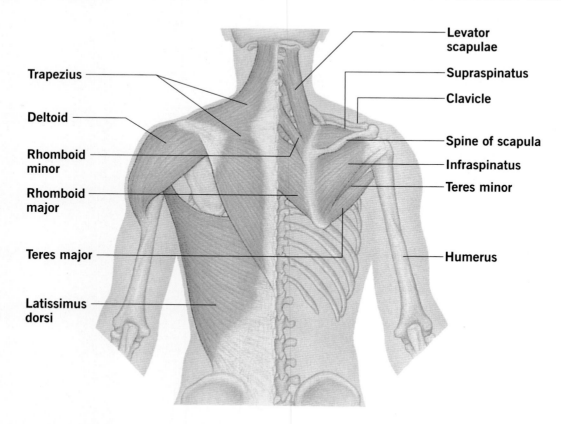

Anatomy of the shoulders and upper back. From *Human Anatomy & Physiology*, by Elaine Marieb; copyright © 1989, Benjamin/Cummings Publishing Company, Inc. Reprinted by permission.

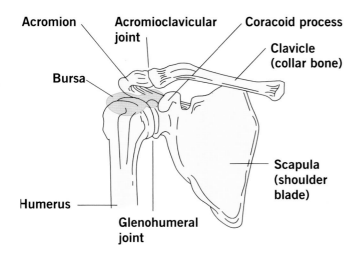

Two of the four shoulder joints: the acromioclavicular joint and the glenohumeral joint.

acromioclavicular joint connects the shoulder blade to the collar bone. In front, the sternoclavicular joint attaches the breastbone to the collar bone, and in back, the scapulothoracic joint is where the back muscles attach to the shoulder blades. It is interesting to note that, although the scapulothoracic joint is not a true joint (bone joined to bone), about one-third of the shoulder's range of motion comes from there. The shoulder's more extensive range of motion comes from the glenohumeral joint. If a shoulder muscle is damaged, the joint will usually dislocate, with the upper arm bone falling out of the socket.

The supraspinatus, infraspinatus, teres minor, and subscapularis muscles keep the glenohumeral joint of the shoulder together and are generally referred to as the rotator cuff muscles. Working in conjunction with

SWIMMING

• If you are a new swimmer, or if your stroke technique is painful, seek advice from a professional swim coach.

• Always stretch at least 10 minutes before and after swimming, concentrating on the upper back, chest, and shoulder muscles. Also keep up your strengthening exercises, especially in these areas.

• If you swim frequently, alternate your strokes so that one muscle group is not overused.

• If a particular stroke causes pain, stop and seek advice from a professional coach.

• At the first signs of an impingement condition (see page 98), ice the shoulder 3 to 4 times a day for 20 minutes at a time.

• If you have a shoulder injury or shoulder pain, seek medical advice. Keep in mind that inactivity of the shoulder can lead to a "frozen shoulder." Your sports medicine provider can recommend a rehabilitation and exercise program to prevent that.

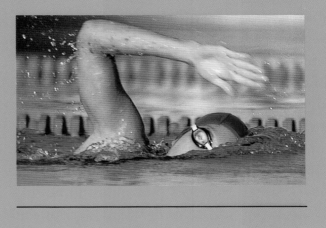

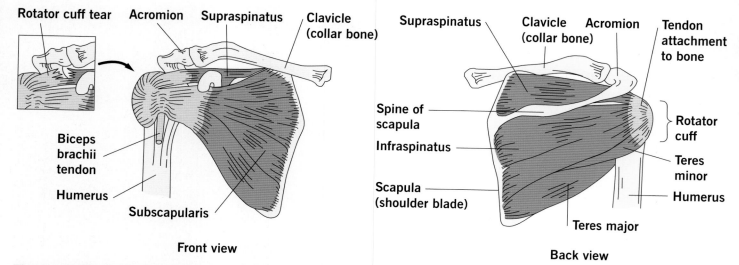

Front view

Back view

These are the shoulder muscles involved in overhead movements essential in many sports. Rotator cuff muscles surround the humerus and are attached to the humerus by the tendons. Contraction of these muscles rotates the ball in the socket (the glenohumeral joint). When the tendons become inflamed, it hurts to raise the arm. In the worst cases, the tendons tear, which can incapacitate the shoulder, and may require surgery. The deltoid muscle (not shown) overlies the rotator cuff.

the deltoid, trapezius, pectoralis major, and latissimus dorsi muscles (see the anatomical illustrations of the back and chest), they allow the arm to move overhead, as in lifting and throwing.

Preventing shoulder injuries

The interaction of the shoulder muscles is complex, since each muscle contributes to more than one single movement. When a shoulder is not working in a coordinated fashion (for example, the muscles, tendons, and ligaments might be moving the bones in unintended ways, or the bones are out of alignment, or a nerve gets pinched between a tendon and a bone), it will become irritated, resulting in inflammation. When the area is inflamed and painful, your arm may have limited range of motion and you will avoid using it. The joint will move, but not correctly, which may cause further damage

and inflammation. Although this can happen in any joint, it is especially important to consider in the shoulder, since its wide range of motion is dependent on proper control.

The key to preventing shoulder injuries, especially those caused by overuse, is early intervention. Any time the shoulder has pain, immediately start the RICE principles (see page 76). Shoulder injury prevention begins with a good conditioning program that develops strength and flexibility in the muscles surrounding the shoulder joints.

In addition, improper sport technique is one of the most common causes of overuse injuries in the shoulder. Always seek professional assistance to understand and practice the correct techniques in your activity or sport.

Acute shoulder injuries are generally due to unexpected accidents, but there are preventive measures athletes can take. For example, protective shoulder pads should be worn for football and ice hockey. Learning how to fall properly in a "tuck and roll" and not on the shoulder or an outstretched arm is key to preventing injuries. Ask your coach or trainer for further advice.

Common shoulder injuries

There are several factors involved in shoulder problems: the wear and tear of simple aging (including misuse), strain caused by overuse, and trauma. It is also very common for shoulder problems to result from a combination of these factors. If you participate in a sport that involves overhead movements and you experience persistent pain, seek evaluation and advice from a sports medicine professional.

SHOULDER TENDINITIS   Severe shoulder tendinitis is an inflammation of a shoulder tendon (a tendon attaches a muscle to a bone) and is very painful. Shoulder tendinitis can decrease the shoulder's range of motion, especially if it affects the glenohumeral joint. To avoid tendinitis, proper sport technique is essential, along with proper stretching and strengthening exercises of the shoulder, neck, back, and chest. Use the RICE principles to treat moderate tendinitis.

ROTATOR CUFF INJURY   The rotation movement of the glenohumeral joint utilizes the rotator cuff, the tendons that attach muscles to the ball portion of the humerus (upper arm bone), which fits into the shoulder socket. Tears in the rotator cuff can result from progressive worsening of tendinitis, repetitive strain through overuse, or trauma. The gradual process of tearing the rotator cuff is similar to a bedsheet wearing out: It gets more and more threadbare until the edges fray or a hole appears. People who keep in shape through regular exercise are more likely to maintain rotator cuff strength. If pain persists in the shoulder for a period of time, or if the shoulder "freezes," seek professional

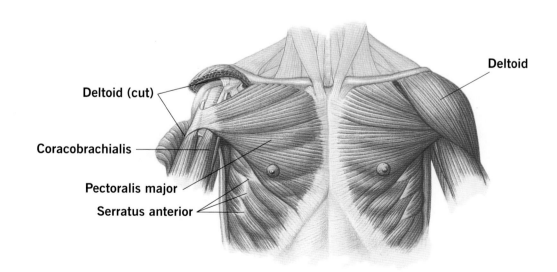

Deltoid

Deltoid (cut)

Coracobrachialis

Pectoralis major

Serratus anterior

Muscles of the chest and shoulders.

advice. The usual treatment for a *complete* rotator cuff tear is surgery, followed by physical therapy.

UPPER BACK AND CHEST MUSCLE STRAINS   Since shoulder movement is linked to the coordinated movement of the chest and upper back muscles, any soreness or injury to these muscles will limit shoulder movement. Continuous overhead activity performed by throwers, basketball players, swimmers, and others can lead to upper back and chest soreness, especially if the athlete's technique is incorrect. In addition, lack of muscle strength and failure to stretch before exercising can cause muscle injury. If you suspect that your sport technique might need reviewing, seek advice from a qualified sports medicine trainer. To care for mild to moderate muscle strain, use the RICE principles.

IMPINGEMENT SYNDROME   This is one of the most common conditions causing shoulder pain. The pain is usually gradual, and gets worse over time. This disorder is a process in which the tendons of the rotator cuff muscles become pinched underneath an arch on the underside of the shoulder blade. The tendons of the rotator cuff become inflamed, leading to rotator cuff tendinitis. The impingement is most pronounced when you move your arm forward and upward. When the arm rotates inward, it causes a pinching of the tissue in the front part of the shoulder. This is espe-

SOFTBALL AND BASEBALL

CAUSES AND TYPES OF INJURIES

• Injuries are usually associated with falls, being hit by the ball, and running

• Most commonly injured body sites are the fingers, ankles, and knees

• Common injuries are strains, sprains, and fractures

PREVENTION AND SAFETY TIPS

• Always warm up and cool down, and stretch before and after playing

• Develop good flexibility, endurance, and strength

• Use correct throwing and pitching techniques. Limit the numbers of pitches thrown and the number of throws from a fielder over a period of time. Seek professional coaching advice

• Wear a double-ear helmet to protect the ears and temples against impact

• Catchers always need to wear protective chest pads and full face and throat protection

• Use sunscreen, wear a hat, and drink plenty of water

• Use protective screening for players in the dugout or on the bench

• Maintain the grass and basepath on the playing field

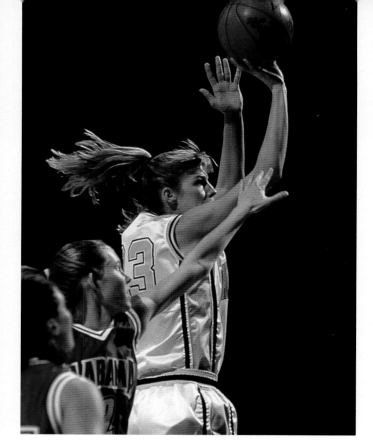

Basketball players frequently suffer from impingement syndrome.

cially common in swimmers, since many swim strokes incorporate powerful overhead motions with inward rotation of the arms. It is also common in weight lifters, racket sports players, basketball players, and throwers.

Using proper sport technique, avoiding overuse, and keeping the shoulder and upper arm muscles strong are the keys to preventing this condition. With proper technique the shoulder blade is in the correct position to allow the movement of the arm forward and up without bumping against the underside of the shoulder blade. Treatment involves following the RICE principles for mild to moderate injury, followed by a conditioning program to stretch and strengthen the shoulder and arm muscles. Severe cases may involve a rotator cuff tear, and surgery would be indicated.

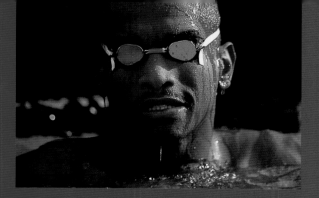

Sabir Muhammad, Swimming

Sabir Muhammad began swimming at age 8 and swam competitively in high school and at Stanford University, where he set numerous records in the 100-yard butterfly event. After college, he was recruited by the U.S. National Swim Team and became a five-time American record holder. He is presently the American record holder in the 50-meter freestyle. Sabir's role model is Pablo Morales, the 1992 Olympic gold medalist in the 100-meter butterfly.

At the age of 14, Sabir experienced a minor shoulder dislocation, but through stretching and strengthening he recovered quickly. During the 1998 summer Nationals he again suffered a mild shoulder disclocation during the 50-meter freestyle race. Sabir remembers, "I didn't pay much attention to it. However, after starting back into serious training, I realized my shoulder was much weaker than it had been before the injury."

Sabir began a rehabilitation program targeted at rebuilding his lost strength through a series of progressive shoulder strengthening exercises, especially the rotator cuff area. Today his shoulder is much stronger and has balanced strength. Sabir states, "I still have to remind myself to do my rehabilitation exercises. Remembering prevention is the best medicine."

99

Upper extremities

Anatomy of the upper extremities

The upper extremities include your upper arm, forearm, wrist, and hand. For convenience, these anatomical areas are discussed separately, but keep in mind that even though your arms have elbow and wrist joints, you cannot move your arms without moving your shoulder or your hand. When you lift your arms to make a rebound in basketball, for example, you use your shoulders, or when you throw a baseball, you use your hand and fingers.

The arm bones include the humerus of the upper arm and the radius and ulna of the forearm. The hand is composed of eight small wrist bones (carpals) arranged in two rows of four; they connect the forearm and the hand. The palm of the hand consists of the five metacarpal bones, which attach in turn to the five finger bones, called the phalanges.

Two groups of muscles move the upper arm. The first group includes the shoulder muscles that attach to the humerus in the rotator cuff area (see page 96), and the second group includes the deltoid, pectoralis major, latissimus dorsi, teres major, and coracobrachialis muscles. The deltoid muscle raises the humerus, which enables you to perform movements such as lifting the arm. The pectoralis major of the chest, the

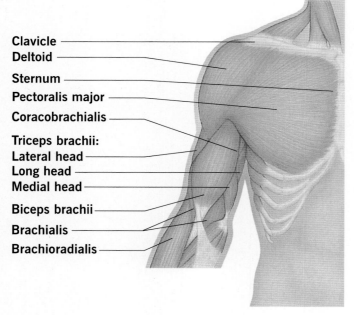

Clavicle
Deltoid
Sternum
Pectoralis major
Coracobrachialis
Triceps brachii:
Lateral head
Long head
Medial head
Biceps brachii
Brachialis
Brachioradialis

Front view

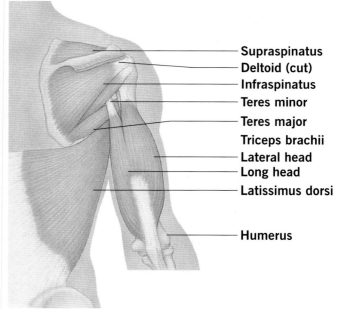

Supraspinatus
Deltoid (cut)
Infraspinatus
Teres minor
Teres major
Triceps brachii
Lateral head
Long head
Latissimus dorsi

Humerus

Back view

Muscles of the upper extremities. From *Human Anatomy & Physiology*, by Elaine Marieb; copyright © 1989, Benjamin/Cummings Publishing Company, Inc. Reprinted by permission.

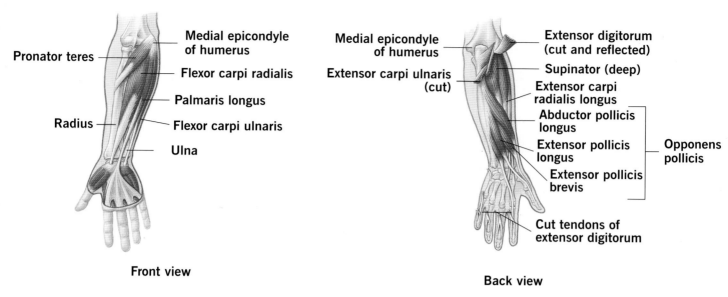

Pronator teres
Medial epicondyle of humerus
Flexor carpi radialis
Palmaris longus
Radius
Flexor carpi ulnaris
Ulna

Front view

Medial epicondyle of humerus
Extensor carpi ulnaris (cut)
Extensor digitorum (cut and reflected)
Supinator (deep)
Extensor carpi radialis longus
Abductor pollicis longus
Extensor pollicis longus
Extensor pollicis brevis
Opponens pollicis
Cut tendons of extensor digitorum

Back view

Muscles of the lower arm.

latissimus dorsi of the back, the teres major of the scapula, and the coracobrachialis muscles oppose the deltoid by lowering the humerus.

The forearm includes two bones, the ulna and the radius. Two opposing sets of muscles move the forearm at the elbow joint in two different directions. Extension of the forearm is made possible primarily by the triceps, while forward rotation of the arm and palm is made possible primarily by the biceps.

The complex musculature of the forearm controls movement of the wrist and fingers. On the palm side of the forearm there are three layers of muscles involved in flexing the wrist and fingers, called flexor muscles. The back side of the forearm has two layers of muscles involved in extending the wrist and fingers, called extensor muscles.

Tendons (connecting tissue) from the forearm muscles, along with three groups of muscles on the palm surface of the hand, permit the versatile range of movement of the thumb and fingers.

Preventing upper extremity injuries

The following wrist-strengthening exercises are important in helping to prevent lower arm, elbow, and shoulder injuries in tennis, golf, rowing, gymnastics, baseball, basketball, volleyball, and hockey. In addition, these exercises can help get the lower arm, wrist, and hand back in shape after an injury. Do the following strengthening exercises 3 to 4 times per week using a 1- to 2-pound weight.

➢ WRIST CURL

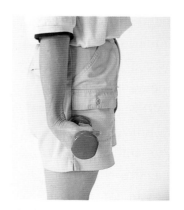

Hold a 1- or 2-pound weight with your arm hanging by your side and your elbow straight. With your palm facing forward, flex the wrist forward all the way, hold it there for 1 to 2 seconds, and let it back down. Repeat 3 times, then repeat on the opposite wrist 4 times.

➤ REVERSE WRIST CURL

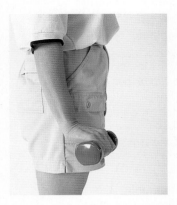

Hold a 1- or 2-pound weight with your arm hanging by your side and your elbow straight. With your palm facing backward, flex your wrist forward as far as it will go, hold it there for 1 to 2 seconds, and let it back down. Repeat 3 times, then repeat on the opposite wrist 4 times.

➤ ELBOW STRETCH (PALM UP)

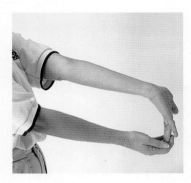

Extend your arm straight out, palm up. With your other hand, gently pull the back of the extended hand toward the floor. Hold for 10 to 30 seconds, then repeat 2 times.

➤ ELBOW STRETCH (PALM DOWN)

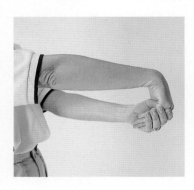

Extend your arm straight out, palm down. With your other hand, gently pull the palm of the extended hand toward the floor. Hold for 10 to 30 seconds, then repeat 2 times.

Keep in mind that stretching and strengthening the shoulder, back, chest, and entire arm is essential. See shoulder and upper back stretches on page 50, and see the chest and upper back stretch and the triceps and shoulder stretch on page 51.

Common upper extremity injuries

TENNIS ELBOW Most people today are familiar with the term *tennis elbow,* or pain in the outside of the elbow. However, this common ailment does not just occur in tennis players. Whenever there is frequent rotary movement of the forearm there is a potential for elbow pain to develop.

Tennis elbow (lateral epicondylitis) involves the tendons attached to a very small bone at the elbow (the lateral epicondyle of the humerus), which attach to the extensor muscles of the forearm, which in turn attach to the muscles that extend the wrist and fingers. Repetitive use of the extensor muscles puts strain on the ligaments and tendons, which can swell and become inflamed and produce pain on the outside of the elbow.

When pain occurs, simply rest the arm and ice the elbow, using the RICE principles. To prevent tennis elbow, concentrate on strengthening your arm and wrist, and use proper sport technique and equipment.

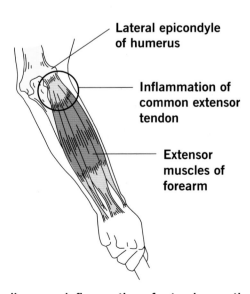

Lateral epicondyle of humerus

Inflammation of common extensor tendon

Extensor muscles of forearm

Tennis elbow: an inflammation of a tendon on the outside of the elbow.

SELECTING THE RIGHT TENNIS RACKET

Rackets are divided into two types, control and power. Make your choice according to your stroke.

If you have a long stroke, go with the control racket. This smaller, thinner racket is more flexible, giving you better accuracy. If you have a short stroke, opt for a power racket. These larger rackets are more rigid, so that the ball pops off the strings with more force, with little effort from the arm.

A handle that's too big for your grip makes your hand work overtime. Grip sizes range from $4\frac{1}{8}$ to $4\frac{5}{8}$ inches. How can you tell which grip is right for you? You should be able to place a finger between your little finger and the heel pad below your thumb.

Seek out a tennis pro for further advice on selecting a racket and technique.

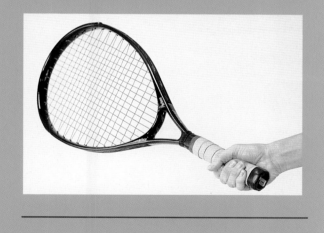

WRIST STRAIN AND WRIST SPRAIN Stress on the wrist can cause a wrist strain, a stretching and tearing of muscle in the wrist area, or a wrist sprain, the stretching and tearing of ligaments and other soft tissue in the joint.

In the event of a simple wrist strain or sprain, apply RICE principles. If there is no improvement in 1 to 2 days, seek medical advice.

Tennis players use their wrists now more than ever before because the game is played with more power and topspin, placing more stress and strain on the wrist. What absorbs the shock of a fast tennis ball? The racket, the wrist, the elbow, and the shoulders. Every time you hit a tennis ball, 6 pounds of pressure are placed on your fingers, elbow, and shoulder. A strong wrist and a good racket can help redistribute the stress away from these areas.

GOLFER'S ELBOW Like tennis elbow, this pain is caused by frequent rotary motion of the forearm and inflammation of tendons attached at the elbow joint. Golfer's elbow, however, involves tendons attached to a small bone on the inside of the humerus (the medial epicondyle), which attach in turn to the forearm muscles used in golf that flex the wrist and fingers. The pain of golfer's elbow (medial epicondylitis) is felt on the inside of the elbow.

Some of the factors that contribute to golfer's elbow are:

1. Poor playing techniques (too much wrist action, poor ball contact, and jerky strokes)

2. Improper positioning of the grip

3. Weak muscles and/or muscle imbalance

To treat golfer's elbow, modify your playing technique. Rest if pain occurs, icing your elbow three times a day. When applying the ice, leave it on for 20 minutes, then

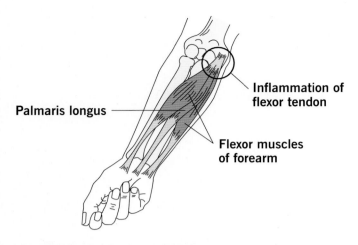

Palmaris longus

Inflammation of flexor tendon

Flexor muscles of forearm

Golfer's elbow: An inflammation of a tendon on the inside of the elbow.

take it off for 40 minutes. Repeat the cycle. Do stretching and strengthening exercises for the forearms, wrists, and hands. Seek medical attention if pain persists.

WRIST FRACTURE   Wrist fractures most often result from falling on an outstretched hand, with the wrist rigid and the hand extended. This type of fall frequently happens when you make a fast movement and slip, as happens sometimes if you are running on a wet soccer or football field. If the injury is followed by pain, swelling, and decreased range of motion in the wrist (particularly on the thumb side of wrist), it should be taken seriously and considered a potential wrist fracture.

SNOWBOARDING

CAUSES AND TYPES OF INJURIES

• Falls are the most common cause of injury

• Sprains, fractures, and contusions are the most common types of injury

• The majority of injuries are to the upper limbs, followed by the lower limbs

PREVENTION AND SAFETY TIPS

• Preseason conditioning and training is recommended

• Warm up and stretch before and after snowboarding

• Take lessons from a qualified sports trainer if you're a beginner

• Equipment should fit properly and be appropriate to your skill level

• Avoid hazardous snow conditions

• Follow lift safety rules

• Stay on groomed runs

• Snowboards should be attached to the rider by a leash to prevent injuries to others

• Wear a helmet and protective pads

• Wear sunscreen and eye protection

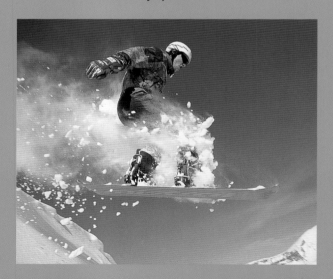

Immediately apply ice and a temporary support bandage and seek medical attention. See page 82 for more information on the care and healing time of fractures.

"SKI POLE THUMB" OR "GAME-KEEPER THUMB"

A fall while holding onto a ski pole or other fixed object can force the thumb back toward the wrist. If the thumb can move normally and there is only mild pain, apply ice. Leave it on for 20 minutes and take it off for 40 minutes. Repeat 1 or 2 times. This will help prevent swelling and decrease pain.

On the other hand, if the thumb becomes swollen, tender, and stiff, medical attention is needed. The ligaments of the joint may be torn, which would require surgery to prevent any long-term dysfunction or instability in the joint. If left untreated, a ligament tear could cause the thumb to heal crooked.

"BASEBALL FINGER" OR "MALLET FINGER"

If your finger is jammed or struck, as by a baseball or a mallet, resulting in pain, or if there is a change in color of the finger and/or the finger cannot extend fully, you may have suffered a finger joint injury. Baseball finger or mallet finger is when a tendon pulls completely away from the end of one finger. Never force an injured finger into a different position because the finger may be fractured, and moving it could cause a more serious fracture.

Start the RICE principles and seek medical evaluation for correct treatment. Usually a splint is applied, and if healing is not adequate in about 6 weeks, surgical repair may be required.

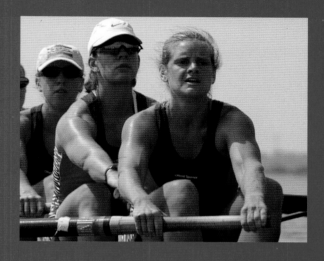

Emily Dirksen, Rowing

Emily Dirksen (pictured in front) is a world-class rower and a current hopeful for the 2000 U.S. Olympic Rowing Team. In 1996, Emily's teams won the women's four with coxswain and straight four events at the Nationals, the World Trials, and the World Championships. In 1997 and 1998, her teams again won those events at the Nationals.

In 1998 she suffered two broken ribs, which she believes were partly due to overuse from intensive training and partly to strength imbalances in her chest, back, and shoulder muscles. During her rehabilitation she kept a positive attitude and took up other activities to stay fit.

Emily recommends stretching 15 minutes before and after exercise as one of the most important ways to prevent sports injuries. She now puts more time into stretching her back and chest muscles than she did before the injury, and she keeps fit during the off season by running, skiing, mountain biking, and playing tennis.

Abdomen

Anatomy of the abdomen

Your abdominal muscles attach your rib cage to your pelvis. In essence, they connect your upper body to your lower body. The abdominal muscles physically support such vital organs as the intestines, stomach, and liver and, along with the spine, support the entire front of your body. Abdominal muscles respond well to strengthening exercises. By keeping your abdominal muscles toned, you will have improved posture and a better sense of well-being.

The abdominal muscles are layered, and they work in a coordinated fashion on both sides of your body. The abdominal muscles may be voluntarily contracted to compress the abdomen during exercise or in anticipa-

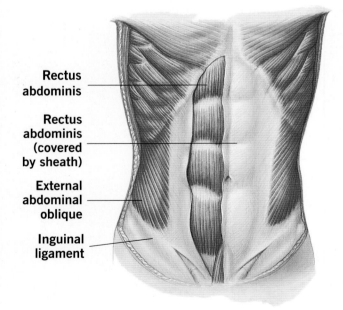

Rectus abdominis

Rectus abdominis (covered by sheath)

External abdominal oblique

Inguinal ligament

Abdominal muscles.

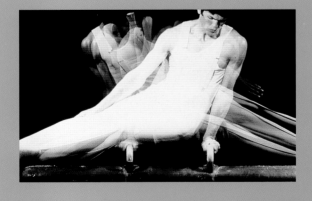

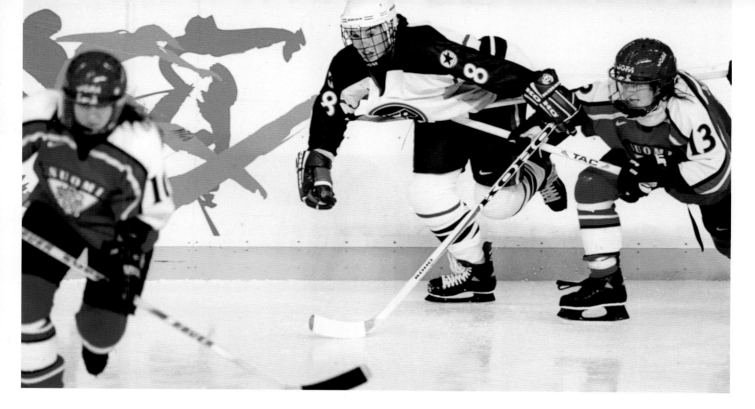

Hooking is a penalty in hockey in part because the stick can cause abdominal injuries.

tion of trauma to the abdomen. When you are at rest, sitting or standing, your abdominal muscles relax and are passively stretching. When you breathe, the abdominal muscles rise and fall. When you lie on your back and lift your head and shoulders, your abdominal muscles contract. Your abdominal muscles are working when you stand, sit, or lie down and when you twist your torso, your head, or your chest to one side or the other.

The abdominal muscles play an important role in protecting the back, the spinal column, and, specifically, the vertebral disks from injury. Abdominal muscles that are strong maintain the proper pelvic (hip) position. When abdominal muscles are weak or there is excessive abdominal fat, the pelvis is tilted forward, and this increases the strain on the lower back extensor muscles, which can cause the spinal disks of the lower back to compress. Although abdomi-

nal muscles are covered separately in this section, you will see how the abdominal muscles are key to back and hip support.

Preventing abdominal injuries

The real challenge is to strengthen your abdominal muscles, since these muscles are always mildly or severely stretched. Refer to abdominal strengthening exercises in Part III (pages 64–65).

Common abdominal injuries

BLUNT FORCE TRAUMA   A blow to the abdomen can damage vital internal organs and tendons. If this type of injury occurs, it is important to seek immediate medical advice. More often than not there is only simple muscle bruising. However, a strong blunt force may cause internal bleed-

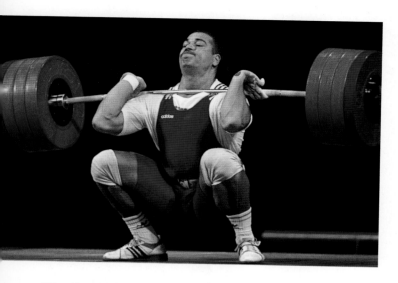

Wes Barnett lifting in the 1996 Olympic Games in Atlanta.

ing, and it is only through proper medical evaluation that this diagnosis can be made.

HERNIA   Lifting excessively heavy weights can cause the abdominal muscles to tear away from their ligament attachment and/or stretch the ligaments, causing the tissue to wear thin. There is then great potential for an abdominal hernia, a protrusion of the contents of the abdominal cavity part way through the abdominal musculature or tendons. This requires medical evaluation and possibly surgery.

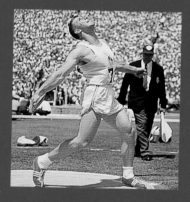

Al Oerter, Discus

Al Oerter was a two-time collegiate champion at the University of Kansas. In 1956 he won his first Olympic gold medal in the discus with a throw of 184 feet. He won three additional gold medals in the 1960, 1964, and 1968 Olympic Games, the last with a throw of 212 feet.

Throughout his career Al unfortunately suffered many injuries, the most memorable of which resulted from a fall that occurred just six days before the 1964 Olympic Games in Tokyo. Most of the cartilage was torn away from his rib cage. His coach advised him not to compete, but he was determined, and he got taped from his hips to his armpits for the competition. After his fifth throw he was played out and unable to make the sixth and final throw, but his five throws won him the gold medal nevertheless.

For four months after this win, Al curtailed all training. When he began retraining, he emphasized overall body stretching and gradually increased his strength training. He also began to work hard on strengthening his abdominals to stabilize his back.

Today, Al stays physically active using a treadmill and taking daily walks. He tells people that they will want to become healthy and stay healthy if they are motivated by a personal project or interest.

Lower back and hips

Anatomy of the lower back and hips

The lower back and hips have the ability to flex forward and backward, twist from side to side, and to rotate, working in coordination to achieve a wide range of motion. The lower back is called the lumbar area of your spine, and the hips are commonly referred to as the pelvic girdle.

The entire spinal column is composed of 24 jointed bones, or vertebrae, stacked from the pelvis to the skull. Between the vertebrae are spongy disks that cushion the bones and keep the vertebrae together. The column is surrounded by ligaments and supported by muscles.

The muscles on either side of your spine (erector spinal muscles) are part of a group that reaches up your spine in three steps: to the top of the lumbar area, to the middle of your rib cage, and to the middle of your neck. The many muscles of your back help your spine bend, and the abdominal muscles contribute to the support and movement of your spine.

Your pelvic girdle (the hips) is your center of gravity, and the spine connects to the top of the back of the pelvis.

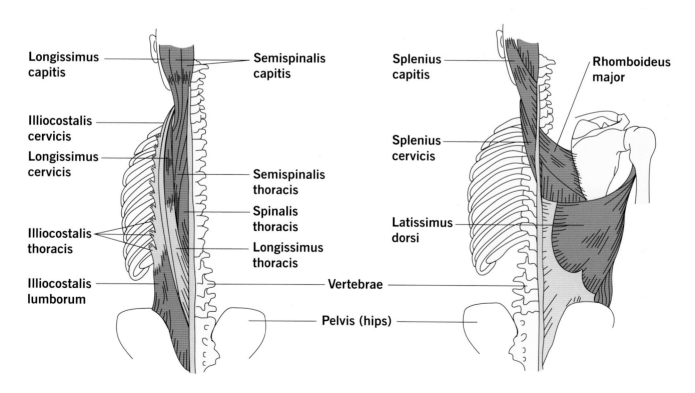

Longissimus capitis
Semispinalis capitis
Illiocostalis cervicis
Longissimus cervicis
Semispinalis thoracis
Spinalis thoracis
Illiocostalis thoracis
Longissimus thoracis
Illiocostalis lumborum
Vertebrae
Pelvis (hips)

Splenius capitis
Rhomboideus major
Splenius cervicis
Latissimus dorsi
Vertebrae
Pelvis (hips)

Anatomy of the back: On the left, deep muscles of the back and neck are shown. On the right, superficial muscles.

Preventing lower back and hip injuries

By taking a few basic precautions, you can minimize your risk of lower back injury:

1. Work on proper posture, keeping the abdominal muscles strong through exercise.

2. Always lift with your legs. Bend your legs and keep your back straight while holding the load close to your body.

3. Sit with care. Sitting in the same position for a long time can lead to back pain, so change positions as needed. Never hunch over. For the best results, keep your lower back flat against the back of the seat while positioning your knees higher than your hips. This may require a foot stool.

4. Control your weight, especially if you have a "pot belly," because this puts added stress on your lower back.

5. Sleep with your back straight, and on a firm, flat mattress. If you sleep on your back, place a pillow under your lower legs. This raises the legs and flattens the curve of the lower back. If you sleep on your side, keep both arms in front of you, with your knees slightly bent and raised toward the chest.

Common injuries of the lower back and hips

The most common site of back pain and injury is the lumbar region. This area bears the forces of bending, stooping, sitting, and lifting. With normal aging, wear, and tear, the vertebral disk material slowly deterio-

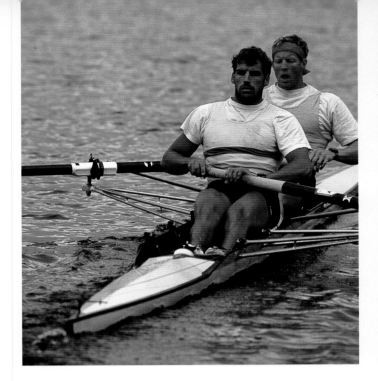

Rowing puts a lot of stress on the lower back and hip, so it is important to stretch and strengthen muscles in that area.

rates. The aging or damaged disk can bulge or even rupture, with subsequent nerve irritation. This irritation can lead to muscle spasms, numbness, or tingling.

Everyone is vulnerable to back injury, especially individuals who participate in sports that jar the spine, such as running or jogging. Those involved in heavy lifting, bending, and pushing are at higher risk for lower back injury.

LOWER BACK STRAIN The most frequently reported type of lower back injury is lumbar strain, in which too much force has been applied to the lumbar spine ligaments, resulting in inflammation and pain. The back muscle responds by tightening (called protective spasm), in an effort to keep the back from moving more and further injuring the ligaments. Preventing another back strain is important because the level of pain continues increasing with

GOLF

CAUSES AND TYPES OF INJURIES

- Overuse and too much practice

- Poor swing style and too much twisting

- Falls on the golf course

- Hits from a club or ball

- Most common injuries are overuse injuries and aggravation of previous injuries, usually involving the shoulder, elbow, wrist, lower back, and knee

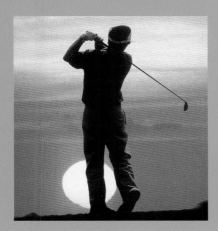

PREVENTION AND SAFETY TIPS

- Maintain general fitness with stretching and cardio-vascular training

- Use proper golf technique; seek professional advice, if needed

- Wear well-fitted shoes and use clubs that are the right length for you

- Wear sunscreen, protective clothing, and a hat, and carry insect repellent

- Drink plenty of water

- Always move off the golf course when lightning strikes

- Whenever possible, carry a mobile phone in case of emergency

each episode until the cycle is stopped. Prevention of lower back pain begins with good posture and improves as flexibility increases, especially by stretching the legs and hips (see pages 52–57 in Part III). Improved strength in the abdominal and thoracic muscles also helps support the spine and prevent injury.

Playing golf can be tough on your lower back. During a typical day of golf, you bend a lot: first you bend forward to get your clubs out of the trunk of your car, then to place your ball on the tee, then to retrieve the ball from the cup. Soon your ligaments, lower back muscles, and spine feel the strain. To balance all that bending and to prevent injury, lower back stretches are essential. In addition, always stretch at least 5 to 10 minutes before and after playing.

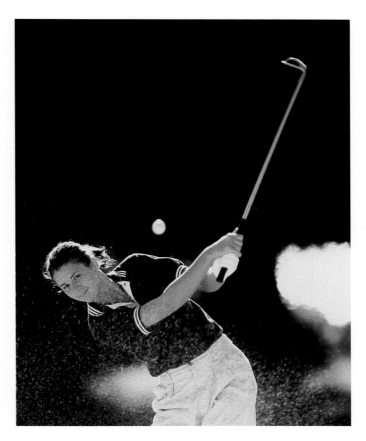

Playing golf can by tough on your lower back.

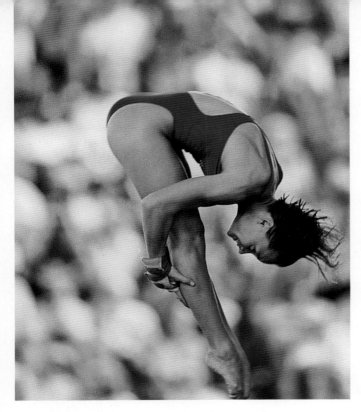
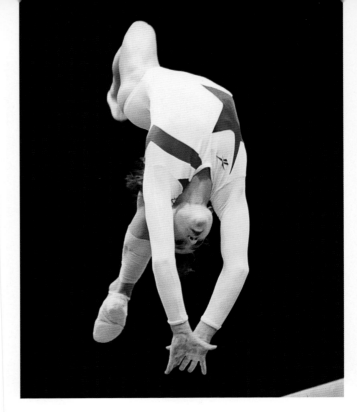

Divers and gymnasts commonly suffer repetitive stress injuries to the back. Becky Ruehl (left) and Dominique Moceanu (right) competed for the U.S.A. in the 1996 Olympic Games in Atlanta.

SPONDYLOSIS AND SPONDY-LOLISTHESIS   When the lower back undergoes repetitive stress, an overuse injury can result. In fact, it happens commonly in gymnastics, where the athlete frequently bends forward and backward. A stress fracture may occur in a portion of an individual vertebra. This is known as *spondylosis*. If this condition is not cared for, the vertebra may fracture completely. This is called *spondylolisthesis*. It should be noted that people who suffer from bone thinness (osteoporosis) are especially at high risk for fracture.

Usually the symptoms show gradual onset over many years of overuse, although a sudden backward bend could also be the cause.

Lower back stiffness, pain, tingling, or numbness from the buttocks down the leg might signal a condition known as sciatica. This is caused by inflammation of the sciat-ic nerve, which radiates out of the lumbar spine region to the buttocks and to the back of the thigh and the lower leg. An inflamed sciatic nerve may not be able to send correct impulses to the leg muscles, and the leg will give way. To prevent these conditions, decrease the frequency of backward bending. Seek medical attention at the first sign of lower back pain. Improve your posture, maintain your weight, increase the strength of your abdominal muscles, and keep the back flexible by stretching it (see page 52).

If lumbar pain occurs, stop the activity that is causing the pain, and seek medical attention. Sometimes rest is recommended, along with pain medications, antiinflammatories, and physical therapy. The focus of rehabilitation is improving overall flexibility of the spine. If a spinal fracture is present, sometimes rehabilitation exercises and/or surgical repair are necessary. Spondylosis symptoms, with proper care, may resolve in a few weeks, whereas severe spondylolisthesis requiring surgical repair may take up to 6 months before the athlete can return to full activity.

PIRIFORMIS SYNDROME   The piriformis muscle is one of many muscles in the hip joint that help rotate the leg. The great sciatic nerve radiates from the lumbar vertebrae and exits from the pelvis beneath the piriformis muscle. Pressure on the sciatic nerve from the piriformis muscle can cause sciatica (a pain in the area supplied by the nerve). Sitting on hard surfaces for a prolonged period of time can cause pain in the piriformis muscle, and repetitive rotation of the upper leg can cause pressure in the region, with subsequent inflammation of the sciatic nerve. This is frequently seen in gymnasts or cyclists. Usually symptoms can be relieved by physical therapy, by stretching the hip and groin muscles (see page 55), and by sitting with proper posture. Medication such as antiinflammatories is sometimes recommended.

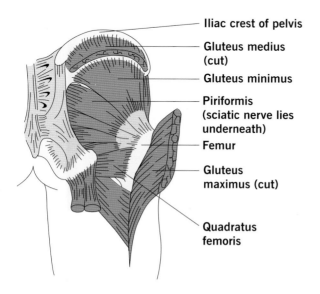

- Iliac crest of pelvis
- Gluteus medius (cut)
- Gluteus minimus
- Piriformis (sciatic nerve lies underneath)
- Femur
- Gluteus maximus (cut)
- Quadratus femoris

Deep back view of hip muscles showing the piriformis in particular.

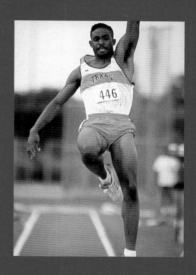

Tyrone Scott, Triple Jump

Tyrone Scott began his track and field career at the University of Texas in Austin. He won the U.S. National championships in 1993 and 1994, and he ranked third nationally going into the 1996 Olympic Trials. In the middle of a jump at the trials, however, the anterior cruciate ligament (ACL) in his left knee suddenly tore, and his Olympic dream was tragically cut short.

Although the injury shattered his hopes for 1996, Tyrone was determined to make a comeback, and within six weeks of his surgery he was running again. He attributes his quick return to beginning rehabilitation early and to a robust program of stretching and strengthening exercises. Today Tyrone follows a daily routine of stretching and stengthening all major muscle groups, with special emphasis on the quadriceps and hamstrings to maintain stability in his knees. He keeps aerobically fit by running and biking.

Tyrone's advice for recovering from injury and staying fit: There is no quick fix, but by keeping up a regular exercise program that fits your personal needs and staying with it, you will see results.

Thigh

Below the hips are the lower extremities, or the legs, consisting of the thigh, the knee, the lower leg, the ankle, and the foot. Because of the anatomical complexity of the legs, we will examine each area separately.

Anatomy of the thigh

The femur, or thigh bone, is the longest bone in the body. The top end joins the hips and the lower end meets the tibia, or shin bone, at the knee.

The muscles of the front thigh are called the quadriceps group, one of the largest and strongest set of muscles in the body, and a powerful extensor of the leg used in walking, running, and kicking. It consists of four separate muscles, the rectus femoris, the vastus lateralis, the vastus medialis, and the vastus intermedius, which lies underneath the rectus femoris. The massive quadriceps muscles fuse into the patellar tendon and the patella (knee cap) and continue with the patellar ligament that inserts on the tibia (lower leg bone). Another important muscle of the front thigh is the sartorius, the

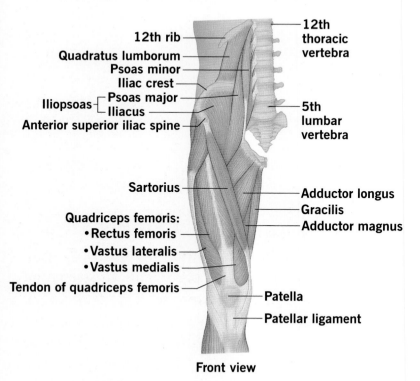

Front view

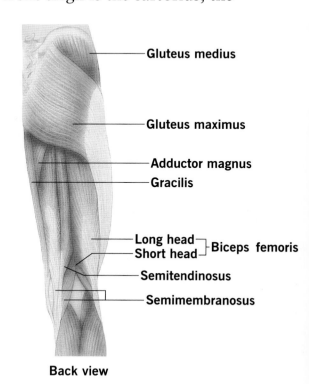

Back view

Muscles of the right thigh. The front view shows the muscles that primarily contract and extend the lower leg. The back view shows muscles that primarily move the thigh outward, rotate it, or flex it, lifting the lower leg. From *Human Anatomy & Physiology*, by Elaine Marieb; copyright © 1989, Benjamin/Cummings Publishing Company, Inc. Reprinted by permission.

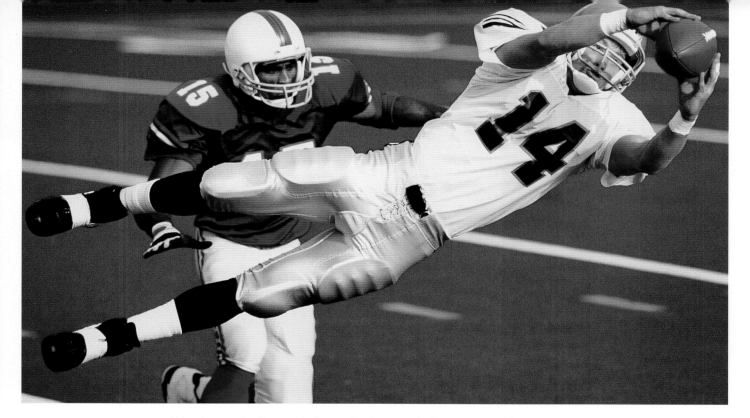

Wearing protective pads in contact sports helps prevent thigh injuries.

longest muscle in the body. The sartorius muscle is an elongated, straplike muscle that passes diagonally across the front of the thigh muscle and then moves downward over the inner side of the knee. It connects the hip to the tibia of the lower leg. The sartorius muscle flexes the leg and thigh, and rotates the thigh to the side and outward.

The muscles in the back of the thigh are called the hamstring group and include the biceps femoris, the semitendinosus, and the semimembranosus muscles. These muscles extend the thigh and flex the leg at the knee.

Preventing thigh injuries

To prevent strains in the thigh muscles, stretch at least 5 to 10 minutes before and after a workout. Particularly in sports like cycling, basketball, or skiing that flex and extend the knee, concentrate on the legs

and torso. Proper stretching of the quadriceps and building good strength in the hamstring muscles will help prevent muscle soreness and inflammation of the thigh tendon that attaches to the knee (see Part III, pages 54–55). In addition to proper technique, wearing protective equipment (such as thigh pads in football and hockey) will help prevent serious thigh injuries. In sports that have a risk for falling, such as mountain biking and snow skiing, learn proper technique, wear protective clothing, and do not take on a dangerous situation. Know your own skill level and limitations. To prevent muscle strains, participate in stretching and strengthening exercises for the thigh so that your quadriceps and hamstrings are in good balance. The hamstring muscle should at minimum be 60 percent as strong as your quadriceps to prevent muscle strain. In addition, in such sports as soccer and field hockey where strenuous running or kicking

115

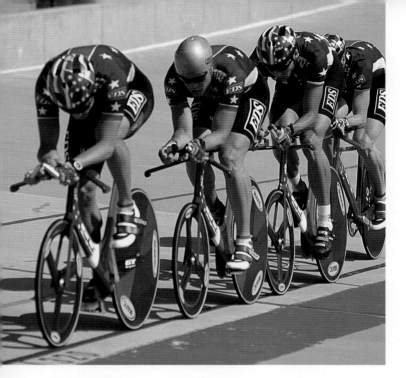

Cyclists have a special need to stretch and strengthen the hamstrings to avoid imbalance with the larger quadriceps and possible muscle strain.

motions occur, the hamstrings are vulnerable to injury. Stretching the hamstring muscles will prevent the tendons of the sartorius muscle from tearing, commonly known as a pulled hamstring.

Cyclists have special concerns. Because cycling relies more on the quadriceps than the hamstrings, cyclists tend to have larger quadriceps as compared to the hamstrings. As mentioned, imbalance can lead to injuries, so extra time spent stretching the quadriceps helps counter that. Your torso also gets a tremendous workout, especially your abdomen as you grind up hills. Remember to stretch and strengthen your abdominal muscles for better endurance.

Common thigh injuries

MUSCLE STRAIN   Muscle soreness can occur with most new forms of physical activity. Within 24 to 72 hours of starting a new activity that has produced muscle strain, the body starts repairing itself. This mild muscle strain is usually self-limiting, meaning that it diminishes in a matter of days, especially if you perform proper muscle conditioning. During this time, gentle exercise is recommended, but if muscle strains occur, get adequate rest and apply ice (per the RICE principles) over the sore area. If soreness persists longer than three days, seek expert medical advice.

BRUISE OR HEMATOMA   A severe blow to the thigh (for example, in a cycling fall) could bruise the thigh muscle. A severe bruise to any muscle can mean bleeding into the muscle and the formation of a hard lump, called a hematoma. This can scar the tissue and cause loss of muscle function. It is very important to treat this injury with ice and rest and to seek medical attention if pain persists. Refer to the Common Soft Tissue Injuries chart on pages 80–81 for the care of a bruise or hematoma.

A kick or a collision can raise a nasty bruise.

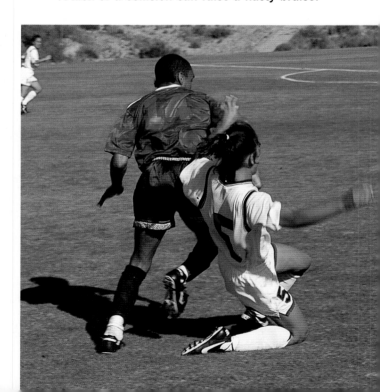

HAMSTRING STRAIN This common injury is very painful, and one of the most debilitating muscle injuries. The hamstring strain can be a simple overstretch, a tear, or a complete rupture of one of the three hamstring muscles. Since all three hamstring muscles attach at the hip and the knee, the risk of injury is increased if the muscles are not sufficiently warmed up before exercise. The major cause of this type of injury is the hamstring muscle contracting forcefully as, for example, when a runner increases speed. Other causes include poor posture, unequal leg length, and over- or understretching the muscle. Explosive, quick, stop-start activities (as seen in running) or extreme hamstring stretches (as seen in gymnastics)

place the athlete at a higher risk for injury.

If this injury does occur, immediately apply RICE principles for 42 to 78 hours. Seek advice if the injury does not improve. Several weeks after the injury, rehabilitation may begin, sometimes with gentle stretching under the guidance of an athletic trainer or physical therapist. To maintain strength in the upper body during this type of injury, and to maintain your cardiovascular conditioning, participate in activities such as swimming that work the upper body. Only when the hamstring muscles can be fully contracted (tensed) without pain can you begin running, and you should continue rehabilitative stretching and strengthening exercises. Always seek advice from a certified

BASKETBALL

CAUSES AND TYPES OF INJURIES

• Sharp cutting, pivoting, and abrupt change of direction cause many injuries

• The majority of injuries are to the lower leg, with ankle sprains being the most common, then jumper's knee

• Hand and finger injuries are usually the result of contact with the ball

• Overuse injuries are the most common in high-level players because of the length and intensity of their play

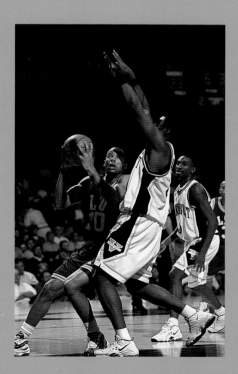

PREVENTION AND SAFETY TIPS

• Preseason physical conditioning: concentrate on aerobic fitness, muscular strength, and flexibility

• If you are a weekend player, maintain a reasonable fitness level

• Always warm up and stretch (especially the legs) before playing, and cool down and stretch again after playing

• Wear proper shoes with good ankle support

• Drink plenty of water

• Be sure the court and hoop are safe to use

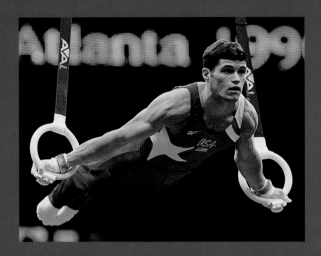

Blaine Wilson, Gymnastics

At his first World Championship in 1995, Blaine Wilson was the highest U.S. all-around finisher (twenty-fifth). He was second all-around in the 1995 Atlanta Invitational, a pre-Olympic event held in the Georgia Dome, and he was part of the 1996 U.S. Olympic Gymnastic Team, which placed fifth, the best U.S. showing since 1984.

Blaine won the all-around at the 1998 National Championships but suffered a rotator cuff injury, which required surgery. He successfully completed a six-month treatment program, which included day-long rehabilitation sessions with lots of stretching exercises and light strength training. He understands that his sport can put him at risk for injury during intensive training, but he is always careful and participates in a well-planned stretching program that concentrates on his upper body and shoulders. Blaine also cross trains by running, lifting weights, and jumping rope.

Blaine is a top medal hopeful for the 2000 Olympic Games.

athletic trainer or physical therapist before returning to a regular activity or sport program.

FEMUR FRACTURE   A complete crack or break in the femur (thigh bone) can occur with direct impact or any strong twisting of the thigh. Athletes who play any kind of contact sport are at risk. Generally, massive soft tissue damage, such as bleeding or muscle spasms, also occurs with a femur fracture. Immediate medical treatment is required, and it often involves surgically realigning the bones and inserting metal rods. These rods can generally be removed approximately 1½ years after surgery, but many times the rods are left inside the leg. Immediately after surgery, it is recommended that you begin exercises supervised by a physical therapist to help you return to activity three to six months after surgery.

THE RIGHT BIKE

Always seek expert advice from a qualified bike shop to help select a bike that fits you and meets your program needs. Bikes can range from basic road bikes to mountain bikes to stationary indoor bikes.

1. **Frame size:** Standing directly over the bike, with your feet flat on the ground, the top tube should be about 2 to 3 inches lower than your crotch.

2. **Seat height:** Your leg should be slightly bent when it reaches the bottom of the pedal stroke.

3. **Handle bars:** The base of the handle bar stem should be 1 to 1½ inches below the top of the seat. The handle bars should be as wide as your shoulders.

Knee

Anatomy of the knee

The knee is the single largest weight-bearing joint in the body. It also provides flexible mobility. When walking, our knees bear

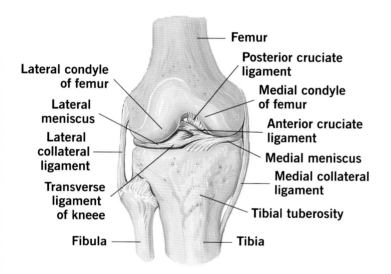

Front view

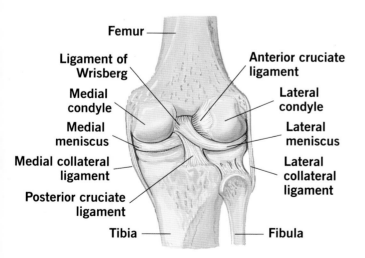

Back view

Structure of the knee.

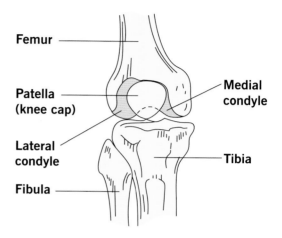

Bony anatomy of the knee, front view.

three to five times our body weight, and, when climbing stairs, that force can increase to seven times our body weight.

The knee, located at the junction of the thigh bone and the shin bone, is a "hinge joint." This means that the joint's movement is primarily backward and forward, but with some side-to-side rotational movement as well. The bony knee is held together by muscles, ligaments, and menisci (cartilage pads that absorb shock). The patella (knee cap) guards the knee joint and improves the leverage of the quadriceps (thigh muscles) acting at the joint. The ligaments on each side of the joint, along with the joint capsule, restrain the knee joint from rocking side to side. Crossing ligaments inside the joint keep the knee from moving excessively from front to back. The quadriceps muscles, which extend the knee and straighten the leg, and the hamstring muscles, which flex the knee and bend the

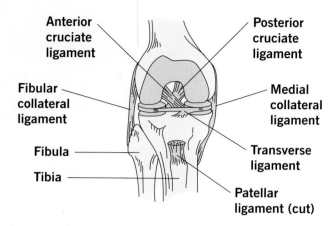

Knee ligaments (patella not shown).

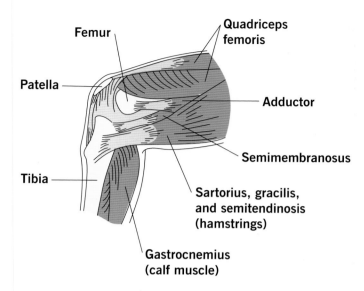

Muscles that help hold the knee together.

leg, together give the knee added stability.

Any number of the knee structures can be injured. Let's begin by understanding the basic anatomy of the knee ligaments. In the center of the knee joint, the anterior cruciate ligament (ACL) and the posterior cruciate ligament (PCL) join the thigh bone to the shin bone. These two ligaments cross over each other. They play a major role in stabilizing the knee and preventing the bones from sliding or rotating. The medial collateral ligament (MCL), on the inner side of the joint, and the lateral collateral ligament (LCL), on the outer side of the joint, prevent excessive sideways movement. The posterior oblique ligament (POL) is located behind the MCL.

The patella (knee cap) is attached to the quadriceps muscle tendon and the tibia (shin bone) tendon. Working as one, this structure extends the knee, a motion necessary for running and jumping. The menisci lie inside the joint and stabilize it, absorbing shock and dispersing synovial fluid, which lubricates the joint. Fluid-filled sacs called bursa are also found in the knee joint

and prevent friction. The surrounding knee muscles, quadriceps, hamstrings, and lower leg muscles cause the knee to move.

Preventing knee injuries

One of the best preventive measures you can take is to strengthen the muscles that surround the knee and keep them strong because they hold the femur, patella, and tibia together and in proper alignment. The quadriceps in particular play an important role in this regard.

When the knee is overstressed, as in repetitive daily movements such as walking or in sports such as running, the knee structure can break down, and injury can occur. Walkers, joggers, and runners may suffer an overuse injury to the knee at some point. Knee troubles generally tend to arise due to overtraining, running on hard or uneven surfaces, wearing worn-out or inappropriate shoes, or structural or biomechanical problems such as misalignment of the

SOCCER

CAUSES AND TYPES OF INJURY

• Common causes include falls, overexertion, overuse, being struck by the ball, and collision

• Adult soccer players most often sustain injuries to the lower extremities, followed by the upper extremities and the head

• Common soccer injuries include abrasions, muscle contusions, sprains, strains, and fractures

• Head injury is associated with heading the ball and collision

PREVENTION AND SAFETY TIPS

• Participate in flexibility, aerobic, and strength-training programs

• Always warm up and stretch before and after playing or training

• Use correct techniques, on a safe playing field

• Wear properly fitting shoes

• Wear appropriate safety equipment such as mouth guards and shin guards

• Drink plenty of water

• Wear sunscreen

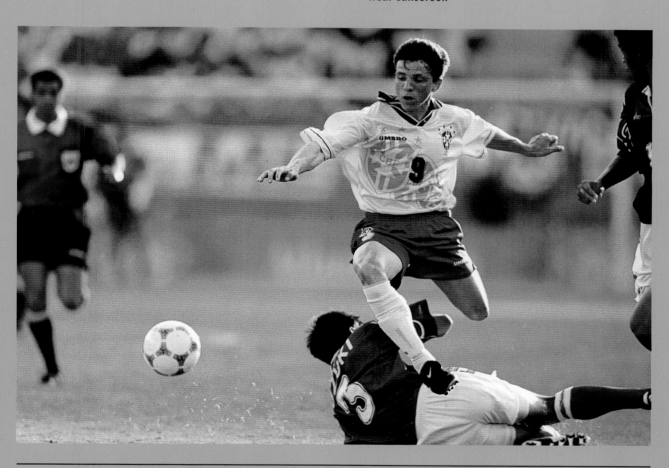

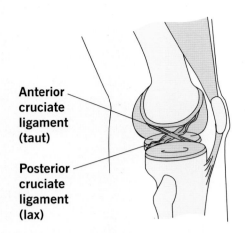

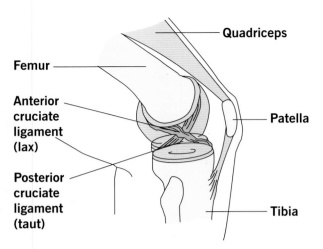

Anterior cruciate ligament (taut)

Posterior cruciate ligament (lax)

Quadriceps

Femur

Anterior cruciate ligament (lax)

Posterior cruciate ligament (taut)

Patella

Tibia

Knee joint movement. The cruciate ligaments of the knee prevent undesirable movements at the knee joint. Left: When the knee is extended, the ACL becomes taut and prevents hyperextension. Right: When the knee is flexed, the PCL prevents posterior slipping movements by the tibia.

leg, muscle imbalances, or leg-length differences.

The first step in preventing serious overuse injuries to the knee is to evaluate the cause of your pain and make modifications to your exercise program. This might include replacing worn-out or improperly fitting shoes, jogging on soft, even surfaces, or reducing the intensity and duration of your exercise routine (especially if you recently have increased either significantly). Seek expert medical advice if the cause is not apparent or if the pain persists after making modifications. Applying ice and possibly using antiinflammatories (be sure to check with your medical doctor first) can also reduce knee pain, although these measures do not address the cause of the problem.

Common knee injuries

Because the knee is the largest and most vulnerable joint, knee injuries are some of the most common in sports. In addition to overuse injuries, the knee is subject to strong sudden forces in athletic activities, especially when it is bearing weight. If the knee gets hit by another player, especially from the side, as occurs all too often in football and hockey, the ligaments and tendons can tear. The ligaments holding the tibia and the femur can also be torn

Knee injuries are common in football.

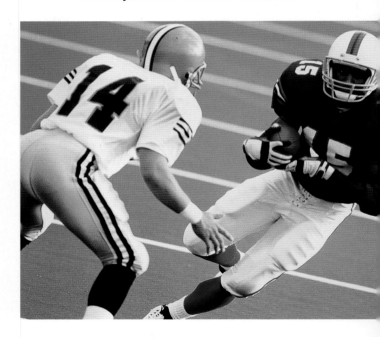

SKIING AND SNOWBOARDING

CAUSES AND TYPES OF INJURIES

• Common injuries include sprains, lacerations, fractures, and bruises

• The most common site of a skiing injury is the knee

• Inadequate release of bindings can cause lower leg injuries

• In upper extremity injuries, ski pole thumb (caused by holding onto the ski poles while falling) is most common

PREVENTION AND SAFETY TIPS

• Preseason conditioning and training

• Warm up and stretch before skiing or snowboarding

• Take skiing or snowboarding lessons if you're a beginner

• Choose equipment appropriate to your skill level; seek professional advice

• Wear proper clothing, sunscreen, and protective eyewear, even on cloudy days

• Drink plenty of water

• Never drink alcohol while skiing or snowboarding

• Follow lift safety rules

• Never ski or snowboard alone or in out-of-bounds areas

• Stop skiing or snowboarding if you are tired; most injuries occur in the late afternoon while making the last runs

when the knee twists while bearing weight.

PATELLO-FEMORAL PAIN SYNDROME (RUNNER'S KNEE)

Pain around the front of the kneecap or under the kneecap may signal patello-femoral pain syndrome, also called "runner's knee." The pain is usually worse when walking down stairs or jogging or running downhill. Overpronation of the foot, a biomechanical problem, decreased strength and flexibility (especially the quadriceps), and overuse are often the culprits. For this knee problem, it is best to cease the activity causing the pain and seek medical advice from a trained sports medicine provider. If overpronation of the foot is causing the pain, orthotics (shoe pads) are sometimes recommended to help correct the problem.

PATELLAR TENDINITIS (JUMPER'S KNEE)

Pain below the knee, where the patellar tendon attaches, may mean that the patellar tendon is inflamed. This is called patellar tendinitis,

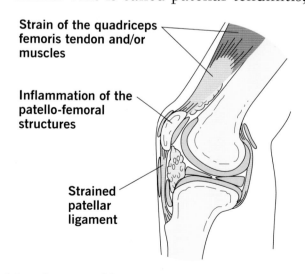

Strain of the quadriceps femoris tendon and/or muscles

Inflammation of the patello-femoral structures

Strained patellar ligament

Injury from repetitive movement (overuse syndrome).

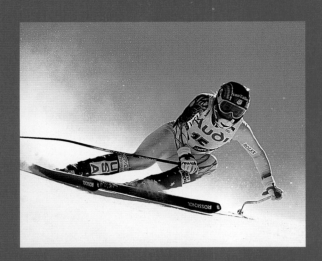

Picabo Street, Skiing

Picabo Street started skiing as a schoolgirl in Sun Valley, Idaho, and reports say she was an aggressive skiier even at a young age. Picabo's athletic career has been phenomenal. In 1995 and 1996 she was the World Cup downhill champion, the only American, male or female, to win that crown. In 1996 she also won the Super G bronze in the Worlds, and in the 1998 Olympic Games she won the Super G gold medal.

Picabo seriously injured her left knee in 1996, but she had surgery to correct the problem and was fiercely determined to recover. With general physical therapy and intense cross training, she returned to the slopes in a quick seven months.

In 1998 Picabo crashed at the World Cup finals, breaking her left femur and tearing ligaments in her right knee. The injuries required surgery, and a plate on the broken leg. She recently underwent surgery to remove the plate and anticipates participating in a well-rounded rehabilitation program. She plans to return to competitive skiing in the winter of 2000 and has set her sights on the 2002 Winter Olympic Games.

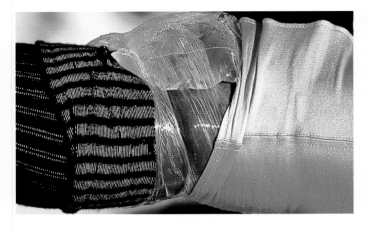

Icing the knee.

also known as "jumper's knee." Stretching the quadriceps and hamstring muscles before and after exercise and strengthening the quadriceps muscles of the leg (see Part III, pages 54–55 and 66) will help prevent injury to this area. For care, cease the activity causing the problem and ice the knee according to the RICE principles. As soon as symptoms resolve, start stretching and strengthening the thigh muscles.

Skiing can put a lot of rotational stress on the knees, especially the anterior cruciate ligaments.

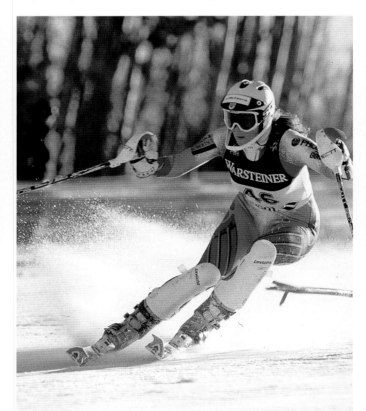

ARTHROSCOPY

Many joint problems can be successfully diagnosed and surgically treated with arthroscopy. Arthroscopy is an imaging technique that allows a physician to see and work inside the joint.

Tiny incisions are made to allow the insertion of a salt solution, which expands the space inside the joint, and the arthroscope, which beams light into the joint and relays an image to a TV monitor. Surgical instruments may also be inserted into the incisions to repair the joint.

Arthroscopy is less traumatic than open joint surgery because small incisions disturb the joint less. Recovery is usually smoother and faster than with open joint surgery.

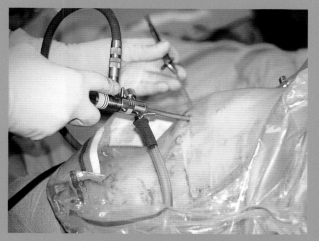

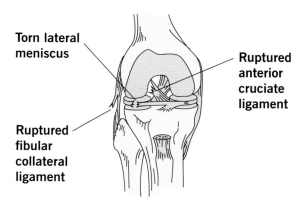

View inside the knee.

RUPTURED OR TORN LIGAMENT
Serious knee injuries, such as the rupture or tear of a ligament, call for immediate medical evaluation. One of the most common of these serious injuries is a rupture of the anterior cruciate ligament (ACL), a condition caused by overrotation of the joint. Activities such as snow skiing, or any activity where there is a sudden change of direction of the upper body while the foot is planted and the lower leg is fixed and fails to follow the shift in direction, can lead to a partial or complete tear of the ligament.

Expert medical advice will determine the type of treatment needed for this type of injury. Treatment depends on the level of injury (whether or not a ligament is torn), the amount of knee stability, what other knee structure might be involved, and the future demand of the athlete. Treatment can range from strengthening the muscles and bracing the knee to arthroscopic surgical techniques and rehabilitation exercises.

Torn lateral meniscus

Ruptured anterior cruciate ligament

Ruptured fibular collateral ligament

Types of ligament tears.

Anatomy of the lower leg, ankle, and foot

The lower leg has two bones, the tibia and the fibula. The tibia is the larger bone and bears most of the weight of the body. The kneecap sits embedded in tendons in front of the lower femur and the upper tibia.

The ankle joint, called the tarsus, contains seven bones, called the tarsals. These have different sizes and shapes. The two largest ankle bones carry most of the body's weight. They are the talus, which joins with the lower leg bones, and the calcaneus, or heel bone, which anchors the Achilles tendon in the back, and which connects to the metatarsal bones in front. The foot has five metatarsal bones extending into the five phalanges, or toes, of the foot.

The main muscle of the shin is the tibialis anterior muscle. This muscle originates from the side of the upper front portion of the tibia, runs down the front of the shin, and attaches to the inside and underside of the front of the foot close to the big toe. Its function is to flex the ankle, bringing the toes up toward the shin. The gastrocnemius is the massive muscle that, along with the

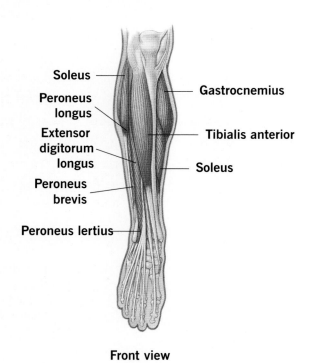

Front view

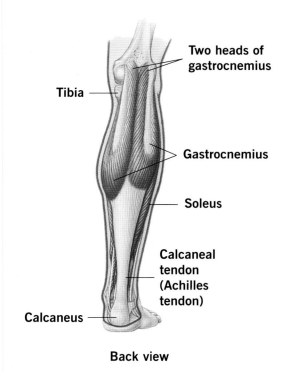

Back view

Muscles of the lower leg. The tibialis anterior muscle is frequently involved in shin injuries. The muscle originates from the side of the upper portion of the large lower leg bone, the tibia, runs down the front of the shin, and attaches to the inside and underside of the front of the foot close to the big toe.

foot

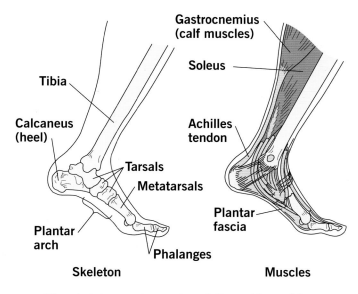

The skeleton and muscles of the ankle and foot.

soleus muscle, comprises the calf. It has two large components that run side by side from the lower end of the femur to the Achilles tendon, which joins them to the calcaneus. The calf muscles raise the heel. The band of muscle tissue along the bottom of the foot between the heel bone and the base of toes is called the plantar fascia.

Preventing injuries to the lower leg, ankle, and foot

To prevent lower leg injuries such as muscle and tendon strains, stretch the muscles before and after exercise and strengthen the muscles (see pages 56–57 and 68). Flexibility in the muscles and tendons—especially the calf muscle—is key to preventing injury.

In contact sports such as soccer, shin guards should always be worn. This will protect the shins from contusions. In addition, always use proper equipment in such sports as snow skiing, snowboarding, and water skiing. Failure of the ski boot binding to release or to release properly during a fall puts you at high risk for lower leg injuries. Always check with your local sports shop for the proper use and type of equipment. To prevent ankle and foot injury, do stretching and strengthening exercises. Wearing a proper-fitting shoe is essential to preventing injury (see Appendix F).

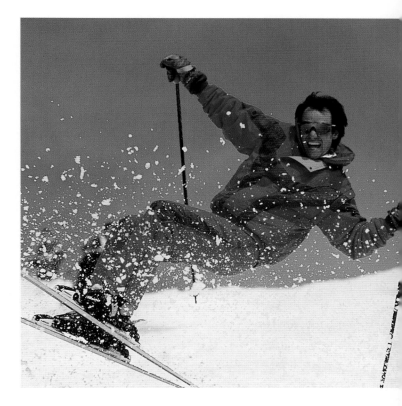

Failure of ski bindings to release causes many lower leg injuries.

Common injuries of the lower leg, ankle, and foot

FRACTURES OF THE LOWER LEG BONES   A blow to the lower leg or a sudden twist or bend when the foot is planted on the ground can cause a fracture. A crack, break, or complete bone fracture with fragments is very serious, especially if both bones are fractured. All athletes in contact sports and downhill skiers are at risk. An acute fracture causes immediate intense pain, and usually a deformity is seen in the area of injury.

Immediate medical care is indicated. Until the medical help arrives, stabilize the lower leg in the position it was found. A makeshift splint can be made from towels or clothing, and ice can be applied over the area. Fractures of the lower leg are managed surgically if the bones are unstable or out of alignment. A metal rod may be used to hold the bones in the correct position. A cast may or may not be used. Rehabilitation of a lower leg fracture is similar to reha-

bilitation of a thigh bone fracture (see page 118).

LOWER LEG PAIN   Shin pain is a common problem, yet its exact causes are hard to pinpoint because it encompasses several conditions. It often occurs when you suddenly alter your exercise program and do more repetitive or high-impact activities. Runners commonly experience aching shins, but they also show up in a variety of other sports such as distance walking, aerobics, basketball, volleyball, and tennis. Running or playing on uneven terrain, among other factors, may also contribute to aching shins. Today sports medicine doctors rarely use the term *shin splints* (although athletes do) because it is too vague.

Repetitive or high-impact activities frequently bring on shin pain.

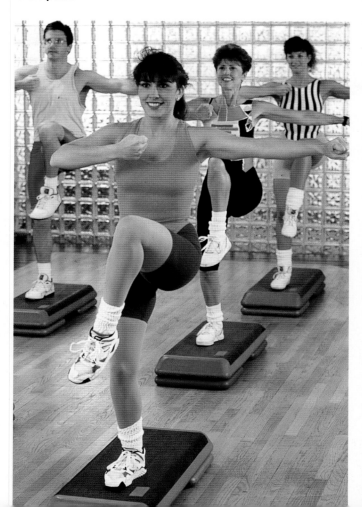

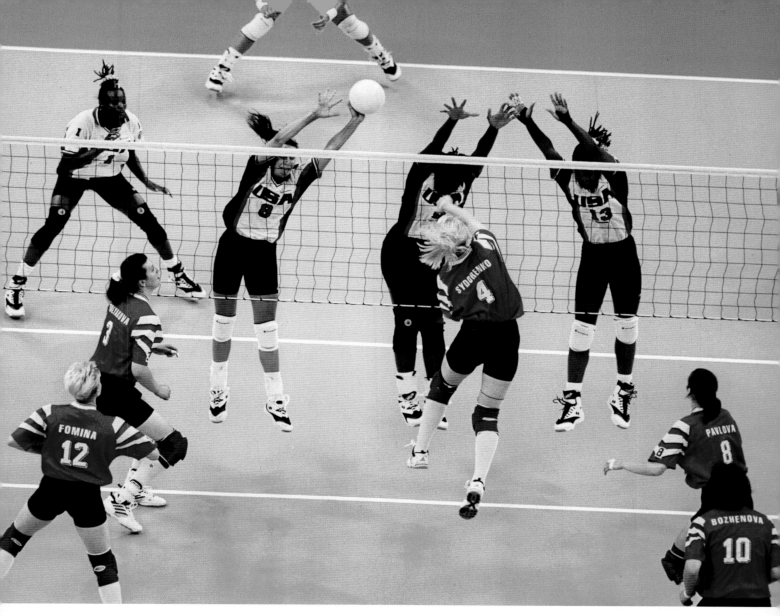

Because of the running and jumping inherent in the game, volleyball players are susceptible to medial tibial pain syndrome.

Injury to the lower leg can range from inflammation of the tissue that covers the shin bones (medial tibial pain syndrome) to stress (overuse) fractures in either of the lower leg bones, or bleeding in the muscles, causing the muscles to swell within their encasement (called anterior compartment syndrome).

MEDIAL TIBIAL PAIN SYNDROME
Usually caused by inflammation of the periosteum, a tissue that covers the lower leg bones, the pain usually has a gradual onset, with swelling at times on either side of the shin. Pain can be triggered by running and jumping activities or by bending the toes or ankles backward. Overuse and the repetitive pounding of the feet are the main causes of the problem. A sudden change in intensity of an activity or sport can also aggravate it.

To avoid the injury, stretch the calf muscles and the Achilles tendon. Wear proper-fitting shoes and avoid suddenly changing the terrain you play or run on. To care for the pain, follow the RICE principles. If pain persists for more than two weeks, seek medical attention. The physician may select antiinflammatory injections or even surgery. Resolution of this problem is short—usually two weeks or less if the condition is caught in its early stages.

STRESS FRACTURES OF THE LOWER LEG BONES   Overuse and repetitive trauma are generally the causes of stress fractures. They are common in aero-bics, dancing, and running. Athletes with thinner bones are at greater risk for stress fractures. Muscles may contract so forceful-ly that they pull on the bone, causing stress fractures, or when the muscle is tired, the bone will absorb the load, causing cracks in the bone that may lead to a fracture. Usual-ly the onset of symptoms is gradual and the pain is intense if you continue to run on the sore leg or otherwise traumatize it.

The RICE principles are the recom-mended treatment. If pain persists for more than two weeks, seek medical attention. A

WALKING, JOGGING, AND RUNNING

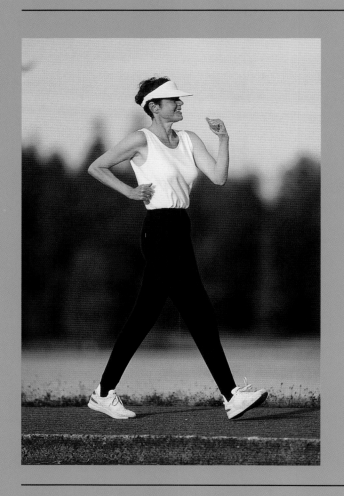

1.   Before starting your exercise program, you should get clearance from a qualified medical doctor to assure that walking, jogging, and/or running is the right activity for you.

2.   Choose the right shoe. Wear your usual athletic socks when you try on shoes, and take a moment to try them out in the store before purchasing. The well-fitted walking, jog-ging, or running shoe should have:

• Good cushioning to absorb impact, especially in the heel

• Enough toe space for the toes to spread as you walk, jog, or run and enough length so that there is a thumbnail space in front of your longest toe

• A heel that fits snugly. This will give your foot stability.

3.   Always precede your jog or run with 5 to 10 minutes of stretching (see Part III). Pay particular attention to stretch-ing the legs, calves, ankles, and feet.

4.   Place the foot. When walking, step forward with a heel-to-toe movement, keeping the inner border of your feet moving in a straight line. Bend your arms at a 90-degree angle, with your forearms parallel to the ground. Concen-trate on relaxing your shoulders and arms. When your shoul-

bone scan or an X ray may be ordered by the physician to help diagnose the injury. Stretching the calf muscles and the Achilles tendon is recommended immediately to heal the area and to prevent injuring it again.

ANTERIOR COMPARTMENT SYNDROME   The muscles of the lower leg are surrounded by heavy membranous walls, which form four compartments. Excess training can cause bleeding within the muscles, which then swell within the compartment, exerting painful pressure; hence the name compartment syndrome. A kick to the shin can also cause the problem. Most often this condition is seen in the anterior compartment (the front of the lower leg). Usually the symptoms appear gradually and range from a mild ache to a sharp pain or pressure in the front of the lower leg during an activity or sport. Movement of the foot can cause pain, and sometimes numbness is present. If this occurs, stop the activity immediately, apply the RICE principles, then get a medical

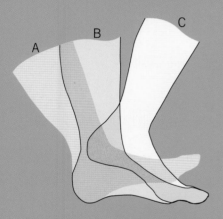

The three phases of foot movement in proper heel-to-toe placement.

ders feel relaxed, your chest muscles are also relaxed, which allows for easier breathing.

5.   Extend the principles of proper walking to jogging and running.

6.   Walk slowly for 5 to 10 minutes before you jog or run. Then walk briskly for another 5 minutes. Gradually move into a jog. Increase jogging and eventually begin to run. For variety you may want to alternate jogging and running.

Listen to your body. Take it slow and increase your pace only when you feel comfortable.

7.   At the end of your jog or run, slow down to a walking pace for 5 to 10 minutes, then stretch again. Remember to pay close attention to stretching your hips, legs, calves, and feet (see Part III, pages 52–57).

SAFETY CHECKLIST

• Wear light-colored clothes with reflective patches.

• In the evening, carry a flashlight.

• Walk, run, or jog with a buddy, or tell someone your schedule and route.

• Wear loose-fitting clothing.

• In cold weather, dress warmly in layers. Because 55 percent of body heat escapes through the head, consider wearing a hat.

• In warm weather, take your walks early in the day or in the evening. Drink plenty of water and use sunscreen.

• Wear socks and remember to trim your toenails properly.

evaluation. Sometimes surgery is recommended. You should start stretching the muscles of the lower leg immediately after the initial stages of RICE, or as advised by your physician.

ACHILLES TENDON TEAR   Tight calf muscles can be strained or torn, or the muscles may tear the Achilles tendon. Tight calf muscles may cause the foot to pronate, or roll inward, excessively. Overpronation can make the foot less stable and lead to all sorts of injuries, including plantar fasciitis, which is an inflammation of the fascia, the band of tissue along the bottom of the foot between the heel bone and the base of the toes.

Inflammation of the Achilles tendon can be caused by repetitive stretching. This is especially common in athletes over 30 because the tendon becomes tighter and weaker. Never continue an activity if Achilles tendinitis is suspected. This could lead to a complete tear. Generally, symptoms develop gradually, and there could be pain and/or swelling over the tendon. Pain

can become worse when you walk up hills or climb stairs.

If you suspect there is tendinitis, immediately stop whatever activity is causing it and use the RICE principles. When symptoms wane (up to 10 days later), stretching and strengthening will help heal the tendon and prevent reinjury. If the Achilles tendon tears completely, you cannot support weight on that foot or place the foot in its normal resting position. Seek medical attention immediately.

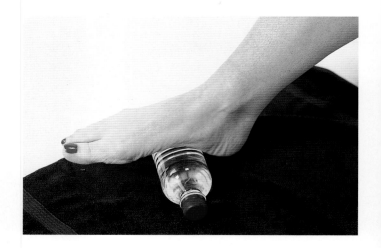

Icing the sole of the foot.

PLANTAR FASCIITIS   The fascia on the bottom of your foot isn't very flexible, and it can pull away from the heel bone when overstressed. This hurts. The pain is usually worse when you take a step after being off your feet for a long time (like when you get out of bed in the morning). The longer the plantar fasciitis lasts, the greater the possibility that a bone spur will form. Pain usually builds gradually and is associated with tenderness on the inner side of the sole of the foot.

As soon as you feel symptoms, stop the activity that is causing the pain. Apply ice

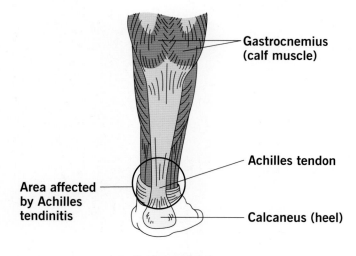

Achilles tendinitis.

Gastrocnemius (calf muscle)

Achilles tendon

Area affected by Achilles tendinitis

Calcaneus (heel)

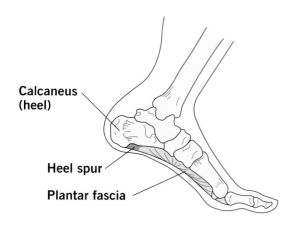

Calcaneus
(heel)

Heel spur

Plantar fascia

Heel spur and plantar fasciitis. Treat plantar fasciitis with rest and ice. Follow the RICE principles for icing.

as described in the RICE principles. Place a ⅛-inch heel wedge inside your shoe to lessen stretching of the plantar fascia. Avoid excessive walking, and remember to wear proper shoes.

After symptoms have resolved, start gentle stretching exercises of the calf muscle and the foot. If the condition persists longer than six weeks despite conservative care, seek medical attention. The physician may recommend injection of an antiinflammatory and/or surgery.

HEEL SPUR   Sometimes irritation of the plantar fascia can lead to a heel spur, a bony growth on the underside of the heel in the forepart of the bone. Heel spurs are caused by straining the foot muscles, by stretching the fascia, and by repeatedly tearing the lining of the membrane that covers the heel bone. Heel spurs can be prevented by treating Achilles tendinitis early and by following the strategies discussed for avoiding Achilles tendinitis.

ANKLE SPRAIN   This can be a tear, a stretch, or the complete rupture of one or

more ligaments that hold the ankle bones together. Most people commonly sprain their ankle when they roll over on the outside of it. All ankle sprains are classified by severity:

First degree: Mild pain and instability with little loss of function

Second degree: Usually a ligament tear with bruising, swelling, tenderness over the ankle, and difficulty walking

Third degree: The joint slips out of place and then slips in again, causing extreme swelling and tenderness over the injury. It is difficult to walk. Second- and third-degree ankle sprains need evaluation by a medical doctor to rule out a fracture. Basketball players, volleyball players,

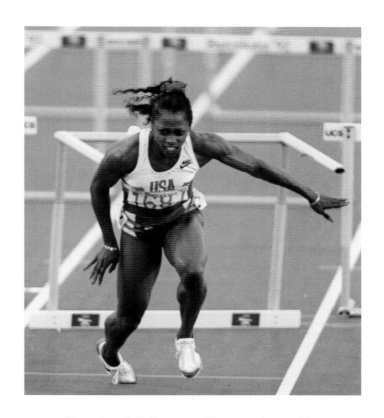

Olympian Gail Devers rolling over her ankle.

or any athlete who jumps or runs is at risk.

To treat an ankle sprain, follow the RICE principles. If the sprain is second- or third-degree, seek medical attention. After a first-degree ankle sprain, strengthening exercises of the lower leg can be started to rehabilitate it. Seek advice from a certified athletic trainer or physical therapist regarding rehabilitation of second- and third-degree sprains. To prevent injury, always wear shoes that fit properly, use good sport technique, and watch your step.

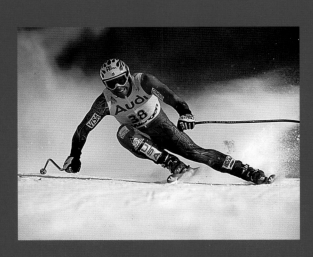

Tommy Moe, Skiing

Tommy Moe grew up in Montana and was skiing by the age of 4 on Big Mountain. He started skiing competitively and soon dominated the junior ranks, winning six U.S. junior titles and three World Junior Championship medals, two of which were gold.

Tommy helped electrify the 1994 Winter Olympic Games when he won the men's downhill on day one. He then celebrated his 24th birthday by collecting the silver medal in the Super G.

Ironically, one year later and on the same course where he had won his Olympic medals, Tommy severely injured his right knee. But this was not to end Tommy Moe's ski-racing career. He still had a very strong desire to continue ski racing. After surgery, Tommy embarked on an aggressive rehabilitation program. He followed the advice of his doctors and physical therapists, which included stretching and strengthening exercises and wearing a knee brace for support. Just as important as the physical part of his rehab program was the determination he had within himself to recover and to return to the World Cup racing circuit.

In 1997 bad luck struck again, when Tommy severed the tendon in his right thumb. Again he followed the advice of his physicians and maintained his focus on returning to competition. He recuperated well and went on to win two U.S. national titles to finish off the season.

He now lives in Wyoming, where he spends his time skiing in Jackson Hole and kayaking, camping, hiking, fishing, and mountain biking in the surrounding areas.

PERSONAL FITNESS PLAN

First, set one to three fitness goals and design a plan to gradually work up to those goals over a 30-day period. Keep in mind that to achieve health benefits from exercise it is recommended that you participate in regular physical activity a minimum of 30 minutes a day most days of the week.

As you create your fitness program, refer as frequently as needed to the concepts discussed in Part II. Focus especially on the four components of fitness: flexibility, muscular strength and endurance, aerobic fitness, and body composition. If you have questions, please consult with a personal fitness trainer or a sports medicine physician.

The following worksheets are provided to help you develop your personal fitness program and to keep track of your progress with your muscular strength, stretching, and body composition:

1. Personal Fitness Program

2. Muscular Fitness Log

3. Stretching Log

4. Body Shaping Log

You may chose to use all of the worksheets to keep track of your progress or only the Personal Fitness Program. Make photocopies of the blank forms as needed. A Weekly Walking Program and a Weekly Swimming Program have been provided as examples of how to use the Personal Fitness Program worksheet. A brisk walk and a good swim using a variety of strokes are excellent, easy, and fun ways to achieve fitness. The more you increase the amount of time you spend in one exercise session, the more you improve your fitness endurance. If you increase your workload during exercise—for example, by walking at a faster pace each day—you increase the intensity of your exercise program.

Personal Fitness Program

Goals

Target heart rate _____

Weight _____

Weekly _____ program for the month of _____

Frequency of exercise _____

Intensity of exercise _____

Duration of exercise _____

Other _____

	Monday	Tuesday	Wednesday	Thursday	Friday	Saturday	Sunday
Week 1							Rest
Week 2							Rest
Week 3							Rest
Week 4							Rest

Remember to stretch at least 5 to 10 minutes before and after exercise.

Schedule strength training at least three times per week with one day of rest in between.

Monitor your target heart rate.

EXAMPLE ONE

Personal Fitness Program

Weekly _____ _Walking_ _____ **program for the month of** _June_

Goals

Target heart rate __175__

Weight __130__

Frequency of exercise __Walk 30 min/day__

Intensity of exercise __Walk up hills__

Duration of exercise __Increase to 30+ min/day__

Other

	Monday	Tuesday	Wednesday	Thursday	Friday	Saturday	Sunday
Week 1	Brisk walk for 5 min.	REPEAT Monday	Increase brisk walk by 2 minutes	REPEAT Wednesday	REPEAT Thursday	REPEAT Friday	**Rest**
	Slow walk for 3 min.						
	Brisk walk for 5 min.						
Week 2	Brisk walk for 7 min.	REPEAT Monday	REPEAT Tuesday	REPEAT Wednesday	REPEAT Thursday	REPEAT Friday	**Rest**
	Slow walk for 5 min.						
	Brisk walk for 7 min.						
Week 3	Brisk walk for 10 min.	REPEAT Monday	REPEAT Tuesday	REPEAT Wednesday	REPEAT Thurs. but second brisk walk is uphill	REPEAT Friday	**Rest**
	Slow walk for 5 min.						
	Brisk walk for 10 min.						
Week 4	Brisk walk for 20 minutes	REPEAT Monday	REPEAT Tuesday	Try walking uphill and downhill. Vary as you like.	REPEAT Thursday	REPEAT Friday	**Rest**
	Slow walk for 10 minutes						

Remember to stretch at least 5 to 10 minutes before and after exercise.

Schedule strength training at least three times per week with one day of rest in between.

Monitor your target heart rate.

EXAMPLE TWO

Personal Fitness Program

Weekly _Swimming_ **program for the month of** _June_

Goals

Target heart rate _180_   Frequency of exercise _Swim 30 min/day_   Duration of exercise _Increase to 30+ min/day_

Weight _165_   Intensity of exercise _Swim 30 min/no break_   Other _____

	Monday	Tuesday	Wednesday	Thursday	Friday	Saturday	Sunday
Week 1	Vary strokes 10 minutes	Vary strokes 12 minutes	Vary strokes 14 minutes	Vary strokes 15 minutes	REPEAT Thursday	REPEAT Friday	**Rest**
Week 2	Vary strokes 15 minutes 3-min. slow swim	REPEAT Monday	REPEAT Tuesday	Vary strokes 18 minutes	REPEAT Thursday	REPEAT Friday	**Rest**
Week 3	Vary strokes 18 minutes 2-min. slow swim	REPEAT Monday	REPEAT Tuesday	Vary strokes 20 minutes	REPEAT Thursday	REPEAT Friday	**Rest**
Week 4	Vary strokes 20 minutes	REPEAT Monday	Vary strokes 25 minutes	REPEAT Wednesday	Vary strokes 30 minutes	REPEAT Friday	**Rest**

Remember to stretch at least 5 to 10 minutes before and after exercise.

Schedule strength training at least three times per week with one day of rest in between.

Monitor your target heart rate.

Use good goggles.

Swim slowly or walk in the water before you begin your swim.

A kickboard or flotation device can be very helpful for support.

Swim with a buddy or have an observer nearby.

Stretching Log

Make a check on each line once you have done the stretching exercise.

Review the stretching exercises in Part III. Keep a log of the dates that you have completed your exercise.

With time the exercises will become a matter of habit and you will no longer need to chart them.

Remember to stretch all major muscle groups 5 to 10 minutes before and after exercise.

Date	Overall body stretch	Neck	Shoulders	Upper back	Chest	Triceps/ shoulders	Back/hips	Quadriceps	Hamstrings	Calves	Feet	Other	Other	Other	Other

Muscular Fitness Log

Make a check on each line once you have accomplished your strengthening exercise.

Review the strength exercises in Part III. Keep a log of the dates that you have completed your exercise.

With time the exercises will become a matter of habit and you will no longer need to chart them.

Remember to stretch 5 to 10 minutes before and after exercise.

Date	Reverse fly	Knee push-ups	Full push-ups	Biceps curl	Triceps overhead	Sit-ups	Quadriceps	Other	Other	Other	Other	Other

Body Shaping Log

Record the date and your body measurements biweekly or monthly to rate your progress in body shaping. At the same time, continue your stretching and strengthening as part of your fitness program. Refer to pages 38–39 of

Part II to review body composition. Measure in inches and use a flexible tape measure for accuracy.
WHR calculation: WHR = waist inches ÷ hip inches
WHR safe limits for men: .85–.90; for women: .75–.80

Date	Body weight	Waist	Hips	Waist/hip ratio	Other	Other	Other	Other

Appendix B

BODY WEIGHT TABLES

Body Mass Index (BMI)

Weight (in pounds)

Height / BMI	25	26	AT RISK	27	28	29	30	31	32	33	34	35	36
4'10"	119	124		129	134	138	143	148	153	158	162	167	172
4'11	124	128		133	138	143	148	153	158	163	168	173	178
5'	128	133		138	143	148	153	158	164	169	174	179	184
5'1"	132	137		143	148	153	158	164	169	174	180	185	190
5'2"	136	142		147	153	158	164	169	175	180	186	191	196
5'3"	141	146		152	158	163	169	175	180	186	192	197	203
5'4"	145	151		157	163	169	174	180	186	192	198	203	209
5'5"	150	156		162	168	174	180	186	192	198	204	210	216
5'6"	155	161		167	173	179	185	192	198	204	210	216	223
5'7"	159	166		172	178	185	191	198	204	210	217	223	229
5'8"	164	171		177	184	190	197	203	210	217	223	230	236
5'9"	169	176		182	189	196	203	209	216	223	230	237	243
5'10"	174	181		188	195	202	209	216	223	230	236	243	250
5'11"	179	186		193	200	207	215	222	229	236	243	250	258
6'	184	191		199	206	213	221	228	235	243	250	258	265
6'1"	189	197		204	212	219	227	234	242	250	257	265	272
6'2"	194	202		210	218	225	233	241	249	256	264	272	280
6'3"	200	208		216	224	232	240	247	255	263	271	279	287
6'4"	205	213		221	230	238	246	254	262	271	279	287	295

Note: BMI is calculated by dividing weight (in kilograms) by height^2 (in meters^2).

Source: Categories are based on values published by the Panel on Energy, Obesity, and Body Weight Standards, 1987, *American Journal of Clinical Nutrition* 45, p. 1035.

How to use this chart

1. Look down the left column to find your height (measured in feet and inches).
2. Look across that row and find the weight nearest your own.

3. Look to the number at the top of the column to identify your BMI.
4. If your number is 27 or greater, you may be at risk for future health problems.

Weight (in pounds)

37	38	39	40	41	42	43	44	45	46	47	48	49	50
177	181	186	191	194	199	203	208	213	218	222	227	232	237
183	188	193	198	201	206	211	215	220	224	230	235	240	245
189	194	199	204	207	213	218	223	228	233	238	243	248	253
195	201	206	211	214	220	225	230	235	241	246	251	257	262
202	207	213	218	221	227	232	238	243	249	254	260	265	271
208	214	220	225	229	234	240	246	251	257	262	268	274	279
215	221	227	233	236	242	248	253	259	265	271	277	282	288
222	228	234	240	243	249	255	261	267	273	279	285	291	297
229	235	241	247	251	257	263	269	276	282	290	294	300	307
236	242	248	255	260	266	271	277	284	290	297	303	309	316
243	249	256	263	266	272	279	286	293	299	306	312	319	325
250	257	264	270	274	281	288	294	301	308	315	321	328	335
257	264	271	278	282	289	296	303	310	317	324	331	338	345
265	272	279	286	290	297	305	313	319	326	333	340	348	355
272	280	287	294	298	306	313	321	328	335	343	350	357	365
280	287	295	303	307	313	322	328	337	345	352	360	367	375
288	295	303	311	315	323	331	339	346	354	362	370	378	385
295	303	311	319	324	332	340	348	356	364	372	380	388	396
303	312	320	328	332	341	349	357	365	373	382	390	398	406

Desirable Weights for Men and Women*

Height (without shoes)	Weight in pounds (without clothes)	
	Women	Men
5'0"	103–115	—
5'1"	106–118	111–122
5'2"	109–122	114–126
5'3"	112–126	117–129
5'4"	116–131	120–132
5'5"	120–135	123–136
5'6"	124–139	127–140
5'7"	128–143	131–145
5'8"	132–147	135–149
5'9"	136–151	139–153
5'10"	140–155	143–158
5'11"	—	147–163
6'0"	—	151–168
6'1"	—	155–173
6'2"	—	160–178
6'3"	—	165–183

*Age 25 and above.

These guidelines, issued by the Metropolitan Life Insurance Company in 1959, are recommended over more recent editions, which provide false reassurance to a large fraction of individuals who are not defined as overweight but who are at a substantially increased risk of heart disease.

Average Values for Body Fat According to Age and Gender

Age	Men (%)	Women (%)
15	12.0	21.2
17	12.0	28.9
18–22	12.5	25.7
23–29	14.0	29.0
30–40	16.5	30.0
40–50	21.0	32.0
Minimum	5–7	11–12
Obese	>20	>30

Recommended Calorie Consumption
Based on height, weight, and physical activity for adult males

Height (no shoes)	Frame size	Desirable weight*	Calorie level based on physical activity			
			Very light (Calories)	Light (Calories)	Moderate (Calories)	Heavy (Calories)
5'5"	Small	129 (124–133)	1,700	1,950	2,200	2,600
	Medium	137 (130–143)	1,800	2,050	2,350	2,750
	Large	147 (138–156)	1,900	2,200	2,500	2,950
5'6"	Small	133 (128–137)	1,750	2,000	2,250	2,650
	Medium	141 (134–147)	1,850	2,100	2,400	2,800
	Large	152 (142–161)	2,000	2,300	2,600	3,050
5'7"	Small	137 (132–141)	1,800	2,050	2,350	2,750
	Medium	145 (138–152)	1,900	2,200	2,450	2,900
	Large	157 (147–166)	2,050	2,350	2,650	3,150
5'8"	Small	141 (136–145)	1,850	2,100	2,400	2,850
	Medium	149 (142–156)	1,950	2,250	2,550	3,000
	Large	161 (151–170)	2,100	2,400	2,750	3,200
5'9"	Small	145 (140–150)	1,900	2,200	2,450	2,900
	Medium	153 (146–160)	2,000	2,300	2,600	3,050
	Large	165 (155–174)	2,150	2,500	2,800	3,300
5'10"	Small	149 (144–154)	1,950	2,250	2,550	3,000
	Medium	158 (150–165)	2,050	2,350	2,700	3,150
	Large	169 (159–179)	2,200	2,550	2,850	3,400
5'11"	Small	153 (148–158)	2,000	2,300	2,600	3,050
	Medium	162 (154–170)	2,100	2,450	2,750	3,250
	Large	174 (164–184)	2,250	2,600	2,950	3,500
6'0"	Small	157 (152–162)	2,050	2,350	2,650	3,150
	Medium	167 (158–175)	2,150	2,500	2,850	3,350
	Large	179 (168–189)	2,350	2,700	3,050	3,600
6'1"	Small	162 (156–167)	2,100	2,450	2,750	3,250
	Medium	171 (162–180)	2,200	2,550	2,900	3,400
	Large	184 (173–194)	2,400	2,750	3,150	3,700
6'2"	Small	166 (160–171)	2,150	2,500	2,800	3,300
	Medium	176 (167–185)	2,300	2,650	3,000	3,500
	Large	189 (178–199)	2,450	2,850	3,200	3,800
6'3"	Small	170 (164–175)	2,200	2,550	2,900	3,400
	Medium	181 (172–190)	2,350	2,700	3,100	3,600
	Large	193 (182–204)	2,500	2,900	3,300	3,850

*From 1959 Metropolitan Life Insurance Company. These tables are based on 1959 rather than 1983 Metropolitan Life Insurance Company height-weight tables because the earlier tables specify lower weights, more appropriate to health-related concerns.

Recommended Calorie Consumption
Based on height, weight, and physical activity for adult females

Height (no shoes)	Frame size	Desirable weight*	Calorie level based on physical activity			
			Very light (Calories)	Light (Calories)	Moderate (Calories)	Heavy (Calories)
5'0"	Small	106 (102–110)	1,400	1,600	1,800	2,100
	Medium	113 (107–119)	1,450	1,700	1,900	2,250
	Large	123 (115–131)	1,600	1,850	2,100	2,450
5'1"	Small	109 (105–113)	1,400	1,650	1,850	2,200
	Medium	116 (110–122)	1,500	1,750	1,950	2,300
	Large	126 (118–134)	1,650	1,900	2,150	2,500
5'2"	Small	112 (108–116)	1,450	1,700	1,900	2,250
	Medium	119 (113–126)	1,550	1,800	2,000	2,400
	Large	129 (121–138)	1,700	1,950	2,200	2,600
5'3"	Small	115 (111–119)	1,500	1,750	1,950	2,300
	Medium	123 (116–130)	1,600	1,850	2,100	2,450
	Large	133 (125–142)	1,750	2,000	2,250	2,650
5'4"	Small	118 (114–123)	1,550	1,750	2,000	2,350
	Medium	127 (120–135)	1,650	1,900	2,150	2,550
	Large	137 (129–146)	1,800	2,050	2,350	2,750
5'5"	Small	122 (118–127)	1,600	1,850	2,050	2,450
	Medium	131 (124–139)	1,700	1,950	2,250	2,600
	Large	141 (133–150)	1,850	2,100	2,400	2,800
5'6"	Small	126 (122–131)	1,650	1,900	2,150	2,500
	Medium	135 (128–143)	1,750	2,050	2,300	2,700
	Large	145 (137–154)	1,900	2,200	2,450	2,900
5'7"	Small	130 (126–135)	1,700	1,950	2,200	2,600
	Medium	139 (132–147)	1,800	2,100	2,350	2,800
	Large	149 (141–158)	1,950	2,250	2,550	3,000
5'8"	Small	135 (130–140)	1,750	2,050	2,300	2,700
	Medium	143 (136–151)	1,850	2,150	2,450	2,850
	Large	154 (145–163)	2,000	2,300	2,600	3,100
5'9"	Small	139 (134–144)	1,800	2,100	2,350	2,800
	Medium	147 (140–155)	1,900	2,200	2,500	2,950
	Large	158 (149–168)	2,050	2,350	2,700	3,150
5'10"	Small	143 (138–148)	1,850	2,150	2,450	2,850
	Medium	151 (144–159)	1,950	2,250	2,550	3,000
	Large	163 (153–173)	2,100	2,450	2,750	3,250

*From 1959 Metropolitan Life Insurance Company. These tables are based on 1959 rather than 1983 Metropolitan Life Insurance Company height-weight tables because the earlier tables specify lower weights, more appropriate to health-related concerns.

NUTRITION AND WEIGHT CONTROL

Five positive steps to successful weight control

1. Set your goal weight. *Example:* Give yourself 100 pounds for your first 5 feet of height, then add 5 pounds for every inch over 5 feet, plus or minus 10 percent depending on how small or large your frame is.

2. Determine the number of Calories you should consume per day to meet your goal weight. *Example:* Take your desired weight and multiply by 10. This equals the number of Calories you should eat each day.

3. Eat three meals a day, plus a snack or two. In terms of food components, 50 percent of your Calories should come from carbohydrates, 30 percent from fat, and 20 percent from protein.

4. Keep a diary to help point out your strengths and weaknesses.

5. Exercise most days of the week for 30 minutes.

Healthy eating: A daily food guide

The food pyramid can help you understand how to eat better each day. Choose foods from each food group, paying close attention to your daily caloric needs. Understanding what a portion size is will help you maintain your desired weight while providing you with good nutrition.

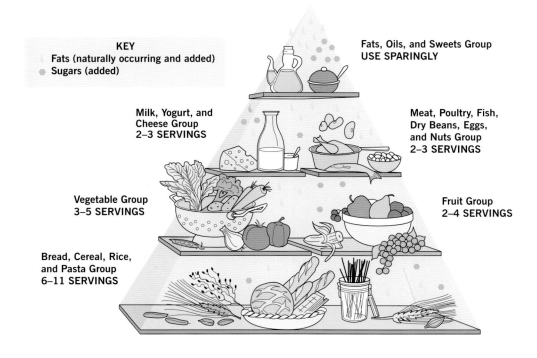

KEY
Fats (naturally occurring and added)
Sugars (added)

Fats, Oils, and Sweets Group
USE SPARINGLY

Milk, Yogurt, and Cheese Group
2–3 SERVINGS

Meat, Poultry, Fish, Dry Beans, Eggs, and Nuts Group
2–3 SERVINGS

Vegetable Group
3–5 SERVINGS

Fruit Group
2–4 SERVINGS

Bread, Cereal, Rice, and Pasta Group
6–11 SERVINGS

Serving size

BREADS, CEREALS, PASTA, AND RICE
½ cup cooked cereal
½ cup cooked rice or pasta
1 slice of bread

VEGETABLES
½ cup cooked or raw vegetables
½ cup leafy raw vegetables

FRUITS
¼ cup juice
¼ cup dried fruit
½ cup canned fruit
1 piece of fruit

MILK, YOGURT, AND CHEESE
1½ to 2 ounces cheese
1 cup milk or yogurt

MEATS, POULTRY, FISH, EGGS, NUTS, AND DRY BEANS
½ cup cooked beans
1 egg
2 tablespoons peanut butter
2½ to 4 ounces of cooked lean meat, poultry, or fish

FATS, OIL, AND SWEETS
Use sparingly. For example, use less than 6 to 8 teaspoons of fats and oils per day.
Limit intake of sweet beverages.
Limit sweets such as syrup, honey, jams, and preserves to no more than 1 tablespoon per day.
Limit candy to no more than 1½ ounces per day.

How many servings do you need each day?

Food group	Sedentary women	Moderately active women, sedentary men	Active women, teenage girls, most men	Active men, teenage boys
Bread	3	4	6–9	11
Vegetables	3	4	4	5
Fruit	2	2	3	4
Milk	1–2	2	2–3	2–3
Meat	2–3 (6 oz. total)	3 (6 oz. total)	3 (6 oz. total)	3 (7 oz. total)
Approximate daily Calorie level	1,000–1,200	1,500	2,200	2,800

Sample menus

BREAKFAST

1 whole wheat or multi-grain bagel

1 cup low-fat vanilla or coffee yogurt

6 oz. calcium-enriched orange juice

Coffee or tea with 2 Tbsp. 1% milk

1 cup corn bran cereal with ½ cup 1% milk

6 oz. calcium-enriched orange juice

Coffee or tea with 2 Tbsp. 1% milk

1 low-fat blueberry muffin

1 pear

6 oz. calcium-enriched orange juice

Coffee or tea with 2 Tbsp. 1% milk

LUNCH

2 cups mock Caesar salad (2 oz. grilled chicken, 2 cups romaine lettuce, 2 Tbsp. light parmesan cheese, 2 Tbsp. fat-free Caesar dressing)

1 piece herb flat bread

½ fresh mango

1 12-oz. diet drink or sparkling water

1½ cups black bean soup with carrots and broccoli (added to soup or eaten as side dish)

¾ cup white rice

½ cup seedless grapes

1 12-oz. diet soda

1 pita sandwich with 3 oz. turkey, lettuce, tomato, and red pepper

1 cup fat-free chocolate pudding

1 thin pretzel

1 12-oz. diet soda or water

SNACKS

1 banana

1 large oatmeal-raisin cookie

1½ cups low-fat frozen yogurt

1 low-fat granola bar

½ cup fruit sorbet

¼ cup mixed dried fruit

DINNER

2 bean burritos with fat-free refried beans, reduced-fat Cheddar cheese, and salsa

½ cup saffron-flavored rice

Chopped tomato, cucumber, and onion salad (with fat-free dressing or balsamic vinegar)

1 cup carrot juice

2 cups mixed green salad with soybean sprouts and 2 Tbsp. fat-free dressing

2 slices veggie pizza made with reduced-fat cheese, mushrooms, green peppers, and onions

½ cup fresh raspberries

Sparkling water with lemon

1 cup light garlic and cheese tortellini with sun-dried tomatoes (dry, not oil-packed) and 1½ Tbsp. pesto

½ cup summer squash with 1 tsp. reduced-fat margarine

Sparkling water

NUTRITION CONTENT

2,032 Calories
15% fat (34 grams)
67% carbohydrate
18% protein (90 grams)
1,309 mg calcium

2,095 Calories
15% fat (36 grams)
67% carbohydrate
18% protein (92 grams)
1,483 mg calcium

2,087 Calories
19% fat (43 grams)
64% carbohydrate
17% protein (88 grams)
1,439 mg calcium

Vitamins

RDA for women/men	Functions	Sources
Vitamin C 60 mg	Collagen formation, immunity, antioxidant	Citrus fruits, tomatoes, strawberries, potatoes, broccoli, cabbage
Vitamin B$_1$ (Thiamin) 1.1/1.5 mg	Energy production, central nervous system	Meat, whole-grain cereals, milk, beans
Niacin 15/19 mg	Energy production, synthesis of fat and amino acids	Peanut butter, whole-grain cereals, greens, meat, poultry, fish
Vitamin B$_6$ (pyridoxine) 1.6/2.0 mg	Protein metabolism, hemoglobin synthesis, energy production	Whole-grain cereals, bananas, meat, spinach, cabbage, lima beans
Folacin 180/200 mcg	New cell growth, red blood cell production	Greens, mushrooms, liver
Vitamin B$_{12}$ (cobalamin) 2 mcg	Energy metabolism, red blood cell production, central nervous system	Animal foods
Vitamin A 800/1,000 mcg	Vision, skin, antioxidant, immunity	Milk, egg yolk, liver, yogurt, carrots, greens
Vitamin D 5 mcg	Formation of bones, absorption of calcium	Sunlight, fortified dairy products, eggs, fish
Vitamin E 8/10 mg	Antioxidant, protects unsaturated fats in cells from damage	Vegetable oils, margarine, grains
Vitamin K 65/80 mcg	Blood clotting	Greens, liver

Minerals

RDA for women/men	Functions	Sources
Calcium 800 mg	Bone formation, enzyme reactions, muscle contractions	Dairy products, green leafy vegetables, beans
Iron 15/10 mg	Hemoglobin formation, muscle growth and function, energy production	Lean meat, beans, dried fruit, some green leafy vegetables
Magnesium 280/350 mg	Energy production, muscle relaxation, nerve conduction	Grains, nuts, meats, beans
Sodium 500 mg	Nerve impulses, muscle action, body fluid balance	Table salt, small amounts in most food except fruit
Potassium 2,000 mg	Fluid balance, muscle action, glycogen and protein synthesis	Bananas, orange juice, fruits, vegetables
Zinc 12/15 mg	Tissue growth and healing, immunity, gonadal development	Meat, shellfish, oysters, grains
Copper 1.5/3 mg	Hemoglobin formation, energy production, immunity	Whole grains, beans, nuts, dried fruit, shellfish
Selenium 55/70 mcg	Antioxidant, protects against free radicals, enhances vitamin E	Meat, seafood, grains
Chromium 50/200 mcg	Part of glucose tolerance factor; helps insulin	Whole grains, meat, cheese, beer
Manganese 2/5 mg	Bone and tissue development, fat synthesis	Nuts, grains, beans, tea, fruits, vegetables
Iodine 150 mg	Regulates metabolism	Iodized salt, seafood
Fluoride 1.5/4 mg	Formation of bones and tooth enamel	Tap water, tea, coffee, rice, spinach, lettuce
Phosphorus 800 mg	Builds bones and teeth, metabolism	Meat, fish, dairy products, carbonated drinks

HYDRATION AND HEAT STRESS

Hydration

Water comprises 50 percent to 70 percent of your body. The cells of your tissues are filled with water, and body fluids such as blood and lymph and saliva are mostly water. Water plays a vital role in physical activity. When you exercise heavily, especially when it's hot, you need to protect yourself against dehydration. Here are some important facts to keep in mind:

➤ You can survive only about four to ten days without water.

➤ You should drink 2 liters of water a day (eight glasses), and during heavy physical activity you need to drink more. Even if you are inactive and sedentary, you will lose 1 quart of water per day as sweat; if you work out or play hard, you may lose 2 to 4 quarts per hour.

➤ Sweating off 1 pound is equal to 2 cups of water. Drink water before, during, and after exercise. Keep an eye on the scale as an indicator of water loss.

➤ If you are thirsty, your body is already lacking water.

➤ Your urine should be pale yellow or clear in color. If your urine is dark yellow, you need lots more water.

Heat stress

Heat stress emergencies			
Heat illness	**Heat cramps**	**Heat exhaustion**	**Heat stroke (serious)**
Muscle cramps	Yes	No	No
Skin	Normal, moist, warm	Moist, clammy, cold	Hot, dry
Temperature	Normal	Normal or elevated	Higher than 105°F
Perspiration	Heavy	Heavy	None
Care	Move to cool place	Move to cool place	Move to cool place
	Rest muscle	Elevate legs	Elevate head, shoulders
	Give lots of water	Cool victim	Medical emergency
	Do not massage muscle	If not better, seek medical attention	

PREVENTING HEAT STRESS

1. Wear lightweight, loose-fitting clothes.

2. Avoid strenuous activities on hot days and during the hottest part of the day.

3. Drink more fluids, such as water and fruit juice.

4. Avoid drinking alcoholic beverages, coffee, and soda.

5. Drink two glasses of water before exercise, one glass every half hour during exercise, and two glasses after exercise.

6. Keep as cool as possible. Avoid direct sunlight. Use air conditioning or a fan to promote cooling. Take cool baths or showers.

PROTECTING YOUR SKIN FROM THE SUN

Preventive measures

➤ Use sunscreen with a sun protection factor (SPF) of 15 or greater. An SPF of 15 allows exposure to the sun fifteen times longer than without protection.

➤ It is especially important to use sunscreen at high altitude, where sunlight is more damaging.

➤ Use waterproof sunscreen.

➤ Apply sunscreen to all exposed skin, especially your lips, ears, neck, and bald spot (if you have one).

➤ Wear a wide-brim hat and a long-sleeved shirt.

➤ Wear sunglasses.

➤ Avoid going out in the sun between 10:00 A.M. and 3:00 P.M.

➤ Check with your doctor regarding medications you are taking. Certain medications can increase the sensitivity of your skin to sunlight.

Self-examination

Look for the danger signs of a pigmental skin lesion, or melanoma. Consult with your doctor if your moles or pigmented spots show any of the following signs, known as the ABCDs of malignant melanoma:

A Asymmetry: Normal moles are usually round; early melanomas usually have odd shapes, and one half is unlike the other half.

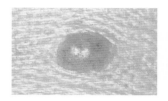 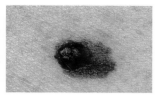

A round mole (left) and an asymmetrical melanoma (right).

B Border irregularities: Normal moles usually have smooth, regular borders, but the borders of melanomas are not.

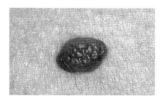 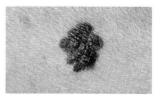

A mole with a regular border (left) and a melanoma with an irregular border (right).

C Color variations: Normal moles are usually a uniform brown or tan color, but melanomas may be varied shades of tan, black, white, or blue.

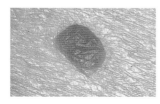 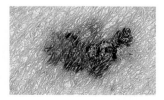

A normal mole with a fairly uniform color (left) and a melanoma with mottled color (right).

D Diameter: Normal moles usually are smaller in diameter than a pencil eraser (¼"), whereas melanomas are usually larger.

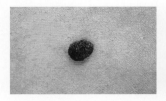 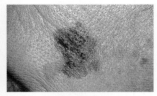

A normal mole with a diameter smaller than a pencil eraser (left) and a melanoma with a diameter larger than a pencil eraser (right).

It is best to examine yourself once a month, using a full-length mirror and a hand mirror, as needed, in order to view your whole body.

➢ Examine the front and back of your body, then raise your arms and look at the left and right sides. Check the palms of your hands, under your arms, and in the creases behind your knees.

➢ Look at the backs of your legs and the bottoms of your feet.

➢ Look at your scalp, neck, and ears.

➢ Check your back and buttocks with a mirror.

If you were severely sunburned as a child, have numerous freckles and moles, or light hair and skin, with blue eyes, you are at greater risk for skin cancers. Check with your doctor if you have questions.

WORKOUT APPAREL AND ATHLETIC SHOES

Winter workout clothes

1. Layer your clothes and wear long underwear. Sock and glove liners of polypropylene retain body heat when wet and transfer perspiration to your outer layer of clothing.

2. Avoid wearing 100 percent cotton because, once wet, it loses all insulating properties.

3. Mittens keep fingers close together and keep hands warmer than gloves.

4. Wear a hat. You can lose as much as 50 pecent of your body heat through your scalp.

5. Wear sunglasses even in the winter.

6. Use sunscreen with an SPF of 15 or higher.

Summer workout clothes

1. Wear porous, light-colored, loose-fitting clothing, such as cotton or nylon gym shorts and a cotton T-shirt.

2. Wear a sun hat with a wide brim.

3. Wear sunglasses.

4. Wear cotton socks to absorb perspiration.

5. Wear well-fitting shoes.

6. Use sunscreen with an SPF of 15 or greater.

7. Always have water readily available, and drink water before, during, and after exercise.

Buying athletic shoes

When trying on new shoes:

➤ Always have both feet measured, and buy shoes that fit the larger foot.

➤ Try on shoes at the end of the day.

➤ Wear the same socks that you normally wear with your athletic shoes.

➤ Measure the distance between the end of your longest toe and the end of the shoe. It should be the width of your thumb-nail.

➤ Try the shoes on and do a couple laps around the store.

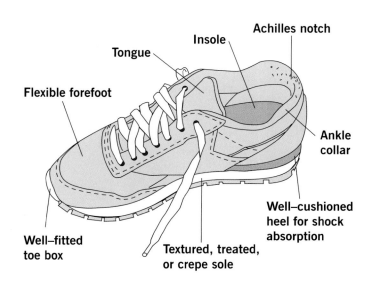

Tongue

Insole

Achilles notch

Flexible forefoot

Ankle collar

Well-fitted toe box

Textured, treated, or crepe sole

Well–cushioned heel for shock absorption

➤ Know your foot shape. If you have a high arch, your footprint will show a very narrow band connecting your fore-foot and heel. Look for shoes with extra cushioning and shock absorption. If you have a flat arch, your foot will leave almost a complete imprint. Select a shoe with good arch support.

If you are considering shoes with a particular sport or activity in mind, look for the appropriate characteristics.

RUNNING SHOES   You need good arch and heel support. Padded heels to protect the Achilles tendon are also important.

WALKING SHOES   Choose a shoe with flexible soles. Heel cushioning is important too.

AEROBIC SHOES   For jogging, running, or aerobic dance, look for a well-cushioned yet flexible sole and overall good support. If you have weak ankles, consider getting the high-top variety.

SPECIALTY SHOES   For specific sports such as hiking, golf, football, and soccer, seek professional advice.

RELAXATION TECHNIQUES

Breathing

You can use breathing techniques to relax your body and mind and to lift your spirit. Breathing is natural and, when done correctly, can help you feel tranquil and focused. Be aware of the sound, pace, and sensation of your breathing, and use the awareness as a focal point, keeping you in the present moment. Try to practice the optimal form of breathing, which is slow, even, without force, and done through the diaphragm.

Visualization

Visualization helps relieve tension and can decrease the perception of pain. This complete exercise only takes 5 to 10 minutes. It can be done anywhere and at any time. Repeat the exercise one to two times as often as you like.

To relieve tension, close your eyes and breathe in. While breathing in, imagine the air flowing up through your fingers, hands, elbows, and upper arms. As you breathe out, imagine air traveling down through your arms as if your arms were hollow and transporting tension out through your fingertips.

Next, to decrease pain, visualize your breath moving up through your feet and legs, then traveling to every part of your body. Visualize your breath going to painful body areas and washing the pain away.

Belly breathing

This type of breathing helps your concentration and focus and increases the feeling of relaxation. Sit with your eyes closed. Take a slow, deep breath from your diaphragm. Place one hand on your abdomen and the other hand on your chest. The hand on your abdomen moves as you inhale and exhale, while the hand on your chest stays stationary. Taking slow, deep breaths, inhale for four counts, and exhale for seven counts. Repeat the exercise as often as desired.

PREVENTIVE MEDICINE GUIDELINES

Today many Americans realize that taking charge of their own health, such as exercising and eating well-balanced meals, is key to the prevention of many chronic illnesses such as obesity, heart disease, and uncontrolled diabetes. It is also well recognized that preventive health care is more important today than ever before in avoiding or postponing serious disorders such as cancer. Healthier lifestyles, immunizations, and early screening and effective treatment of disease are the cornerstones of preventive medicine.

Because preventive medicine has also never been more complex, leading medical authorities have reached basic agreement on a timeline for tests, immunizations, and examinations to be administered to adults age 19 and older. The following chart presents these recommendations. Please determine from the chart what care you may need, then check with your physician about implementing it.

Preventive Medicine Guidelines

Men and women	Ages 19 to 49	Ages 50 to 64	Age 65 and over
Periodic health exam	At intervals recommended by your doctor		
Blood pressure/weight	Every 2 years		
Height	Periodically		
Vision exam			Periodically by wall chart
Hearing exam			Periodically by hearing history
Cholesterol test	Every 5 years	Every 5 years	Optional
Rectal exam		Every year	Every year
FOBT (stool sample)		Every year	Every year
Sigmoidoscopy[1]		Every 3 to 5 years	Every 3 to 5 years
Measles/mumps/rubella (MMR) immunization	For those born after 1956 with no history of having the diseases		
Tuberculin test	Once during a lifetime for those age 35 or younger		
Tetanus/diphtheria immunization		Every 10 years	
Influenza immunization			Every year
Pneumococcal immunization			Once

Women only	Ages 18 to 39	Ages 40 to 49	Ages 50 to 64	Age 65 and over
Pap smear	At least every 3 years if sexually active and cervix present[2]			
Clinical breast exam		Every year	Every year	Every year
Mammogram		Every 1 to 2 years	Every 1 to 2 years	Every 1 to 2 years
Rubella immunization[3]	Once for women of child-bearing age			

1. If recommended by your doctor.
2. If sexual history is in question, begin Pap smears at age 18. Chlamydia screening is indicated for all sexually active women age 20 and younger. May stop at age 65 if previous Pap smears were consistently negative.
3. Unless documented evidence of prior vaccination or positive serologic status.

PREVENTING INFECTIONS TRANSMITTED BY BLOOD

Infectious diseases, or diseases that can spread from one person to another, are caused by microorganisms, or germs. These disease-causing germs may be present in human blood and certain bodily fluids.

The most common germs are bacteria and viruses. Blood could be infected with bacteria that is normally found on the skin, for example, but bacterial infections respond to antibiotic treatment. However, if blood is infected with a virus such as hepatitis A, B, C, or D (which may cause liver disease) or HIV (which causes AIDS), treatment is more difficult, since antibiotics do not work on viruses.

Prevention therefore is critical. Vaccines are currently available for hepatitis A and B to help prevent disease if a person is exposed to those viruses. However, these vaccines are usually given *before* exposure.

Universal precautions, as they are called, have been developed for the care of someone who is bleeding in order to prevent possible infection by germs in their blood. These precautions take the approach that all blood and certain bodily fluids in these cases should be treated as if they are known to be infected. By understanding and following these precautions, you will decrease your risk for contagion when caring for a bleeding athlete.

Universal precautions

➢ Use personal protective equipment such as latex gloves, a clean, dry cloth, or a face shield whenever possible.

➢ Avoid contact with bodily fluids and blood if at all possible.

➢ Keep open wounds covered with a dressing to prevent exposure to another person's blood.

➢ Always wash your hands with soap and water before and after giving care.

➢ Avoid touching objects soiled with bodily fluids and/or blood. Bag and seal items for proper disposal, and dispose of items while wearing protection.

RESOURCES

Sports and fitness organizations

Amateur Athletic Union (AAU)
The Walt Disney Resort
P.O. Box 10000
Lake Buena Vista, FL 32830
Ph: (407) 363-6170
Fax: (407) 363-6710

American Alliance for Health, Physical
Education, Recreation and Dance
(AAHPERD)
1900 Association Drive
Reston, VA 22091
Ph: (703) 476-3400
Fax: (703) 476-9527

American College of Sports Medicine (ACSM)
401 West Michigan Street
Indianapolis, IN 46206-1440
Ph: (327) 637-9200
Fax: (317) 634-7817

Boys and Girls Clubs of America
1230 W. Peachtree Street., N.W.
Atlanta, GA 30309
Ph: (404) 815-5700
Fax: (404) 815-5789

Catholic Youth Organization (CYO)
1011 First Avenue, Room 620
New York, NY 10022
Ph: (212) 371-1000
Fax: (212) 371-1000, ext. 3465

Jewish Community Centers Association
15 East 26th Street, Suite 1417
New York, NY 10010
Ph: (212) 532-4949
Fax: (212) 481-4174

National Association of Police Athletic
Leagues, Inc.
618 North U.S. Hwy. 1, Suite 201
North Palm Beach, FL 33406
Ph: (407) 844-1823
Fax: (407) 863-6120
e-mail: copnkid1@aol.com

National Associations for Sport and Physical
Education (NASPE)
P.O. Box 704
Walford, MD 20604
Ph: (800) 321-0789
Fax: (703) 476-9527

National Congress of State Games
P.O. Box 7138
401 North 31st Street
Room 620
Billings, MT 59103
Ph: (406) 254-7426
Fax: (406) 254-7439
e-mail: NCSG@aol.com

National Exploring Division, Boy Scouts of
America
1325 West Walnut Hill Lane
Irving, TX 75038
Ph: (214) 580-2423
Fax: (214) 580-2502

Native American Sports Council
1765 South 8th Street
Suite T-6
Colorado Springs, CO 80906
Ph: (719) 527-8511
Fax: (719) 527-1649

President's Council on Physical Fitness
450 5th Street, N.W., Suite 7103
Washington, DC 20001
Ph: (202) 272-3424

Shape Up America!
6707 Democracy Blvd., Suite 306
Bethesda, MD 20817
http://www.shapeup.org/

U.S. National Senior Sports Organization
12520 Olive Blvd.
St. Louis, MO 63141
Ph: (314) 621-5545
Fax: (314) 621-5536

YMCA of the USA
101 North Wacker Drive
Chicago, IL 60606
Ph: (312) 977-0031
Fax: (312) 977-9063

YWCA of the USA
726 Broadway, 5th Floor
New York, NY 10003
Ph: (212) 614-2700
Fax: (212) 677-9716

Health and disease prevention

American Cancer Society
Ph: (800) ACS-2245
Website: http://www.cancer.org

American Dietetic Association
216 W. Jackson Blvd., Suite 800
Chicago, IL 60606-6995
Ph: (312) 899-0040 or (800) 366-1655

American Heart Association
7320 Greenville Avenue
Dallas, TX 75231
Ph: (800) 233-1230

Arthritis Foundation National Office
1330 West Peachtree Street
Atlanta, GA 30309
Ph: (404) 872-7100
Website: http://www.arthritis.org

Centers for Disease Control and Prevention
1600 Clifton Rd., N.E.
Atlanta, GA 30333
Ph: (404) 639-3311 or (800) 311-3435
Website: http://www.cdc.gov/

National Cancer Institute (NCI)
Ph: (800-422-6237)
Website: http://www.nci.nih.gov

The National Health Information Center
   (NHIC)
Referral Specialist
P.O. Box 1133
Washington, DC 20013-1133
Ph: (800) 336-4797
Fax: (301) 984-4256

National Heart, Lung, and Blood Institute
4733 Bethesda Avenue, Suite 530
Bethesda, MD 20814
Ph: (301) 951-3260

National Heart, Lung, and Blood Institute
   Information Center
P.O. Box 30105
Bethesda, MD 20824-0105
Ph: (301) 251-1222
Fax: (301) 251-1223
Website: http://www.nhlbi.nih.gov/nhlbi
   /nhlbi.htm

National Institute of Health
Health Promotion Resource Center
Stanford Center for Research in Disease
   Prevention
100 Welch Road
Palo Alto, CA 94304-1885
Ph: (415) 723-0003

National Institute of Mental Health
5600 Fishers Lane, Rm. 7C-02, MSC 8030
Bethesda, MD 20892-8030
Ph: (301) 443-4513
Fax: (301) 443-4279
Website: http://www.nimh.nih.gov/

National Institute on Aging
Building 31, Room 5C27
31 Center Drive, MSC 2292
Bethesda, MD 20892-2292
Ph: (301) 496-1752
Website: http://www.nih.gov/nia/

Office of Disease Prevention and Health
    Promotion
Ph: (800) 336-4797
Website: http://www.odphp.osophs.dhhs.gov/

U.S. Olympic Committee

Public Information and Media Relations
    Division
One Olympic Plaza
Colorado Springs, CO 80909
Ph: (719) 578-4529
Fax: (719) 578-4677

U.S. Olympic Training Centers
One Olympic Plaza
Colorado Springs, CO 80909
Ph: (719) 578-4501
Fax: (719) 578-4645

Colorado Springs USOTC
One Olympic Plaza
Colorado Spings, CO 80909
Ph. (719) 578-1500, ext. 5500
Fax: (719) 632-1035

Lake Placid USOTC
421 Old Military Road
Lake Placid, NY 12946
Ph: (518) 523-2600
Fax: (518) 523-1370

Arco USOTC Training Center
1750 Wueste Road
Chula Vista, CA 91915
Ph: (619) 656-1300
Fax: (619) 482-6200

U.S. Olympic Education Center
c/o Northern Michigan University
Marquette, MI 49855
Ph: (916) 227-2888
Fax: (916) 227-2848

USOC-affiliated sports organizations

Archery
National Archery Association
One Olympic Plaza
Colorado Springs, CO 90909
Ph: (719) 578-1376
Fax: (719) 632-1738
Website: http://www.USAchery.org
e-mail: naa@USArchery.org

Badminton
USA Badminton
One Olympic Plaza
Colorado Springs, CO 80909
Ph: (719) 578-4808
Fax: (719) 578-4507
Website: http://www.mid).external.hp.com/
    stanb/usba/usba.html
e-mail: USBA1996@aol.com

Baseball
USA Baseball
2100 Greenwood Avenue
Trenton, NJ 08609
Ph: (609) 586-2381
Fax: (609) 587-1818
Website: http://www.usabaseball.com

Basketball
USA Basketball
5465 Mark Dabling Blvd.
Colorado Springs, CO 80918
Ph: (719) 590-4800
Fax: (719) 590-4811
Website: http://www.usabasketball.com

Biathlon
U.S. Biathlon Association
P.O. Box 297
29 Church Street
Lower Level #5
Burlington, VT 05402
Ph: (802) 862-0338
Fax: (802) 862-0443
e-mail: USBiathlon@aol.com

Bobsled
U.S. Bobsled and Skeleton Federation
P.O. Box 828
421 Old Military Road
Lake Placid, NY 12946
Ph: (518) 523-1842
Fax: (518) 523-9491
Website: http://www.sir-tech.com/bobsled
e-mail: info@usabobsled.org

Boxing
USA Boxing
One Olympic Plaza
Colorado Springs, CO 80909
Ph: (719) 578-4506
Fax: (719) 632-3426
e-mail: USABoxing@aol.com

Canoeing/Kayaking
American Canoe Association
7432 Alban Station Blvd.
Suite B-226
Springfield, VA 22150
Ph: (703) 451-0141
Fax: (703) 451-2245
Website: http://www.usacanoekayak.org
e-mail: USCKT@aol.com

Curling
USA Curling
P.O. Box 866
1100 Center Point Drive
Stevens Point, WI 54481
Ph: (715) 341-1199
Fax: (715) 344-6885
Website: http://www.coredes.com/-usacurl
e-mail: usacurl@coredes.com

Cycling
USA Cycling, Inc.
One Olympic Plaza
Colorado Springs, CO 80909
Ph: (719) 578-4581
Fax: (719) 578-4596
Website: http://www.usacycling.org

Diving
United States Diving, Inc.
Pan American Plaza
Suite 430
201 South Capitol Avenue
Indianapolis, IN 46225
Ph: (317) 237-5252
Fax: (317) 237-5257

Equestrian
American Horse Shows Association
220 East 42nd Street
Suite 409
New York, NY 10017
Ph: (212) 972-2472
Fax: (212) 983-7286
e-mail: Britches@ix.netcom.com

Fencing
U.S. Fencing Association
One Olympic Plaza
Colorado Springs, CO 80909
Ph: (719) 578-4511
Fax: (719) 632-5737
Website: http://www.usfa.org
e-mail: USFencing@aol.com

Field Hockey
U.S. Field Hockey Association
One Olympic Plaza
Colorado Springs, CO 80909
Ph: (719) 578-4567
Fax: (719) 632-0979
Website: http://www.inovatec.com/usfha
e-mail: USFieldHoc@aol.com

Figure Skating
U.S. Figure Skating Association
20 First Street
Colorado Springs, CO 80906
Ph: (719) 635-5200
Fax: (719)635-9548
Website: http://aolsports.com/Grandstand/
   USFSA/index.htm
e-mail: USFA1@aol.com

Gymnastics
USA Gymnastics
Pan American Plaza
Suite 300
201 South Capitol Avenue
Indianpolis, IN 46325
Ph: (317) 237-5050
Fax: (317) 237-5069
Website: http://www.usa-gymnastics.org/usag

Ice Hockey
USA Hockey, Inc.
1715 Bob Johnson Road
Colorado Springs, CO 80906
Ph: (719) 599-5500
Fax: (719) 599-5994
Website: http://www.usahockey.com
e-mail: usah@usahockey.org

Judo
United States Judo, Inc.
One Olympic Plaza
Colorado Springs, CO 80909
Ph: (719) 578-4730
Fax: (719) 578-4733
Website: http://www.usjudo.org

Luge
U.S. Luge Association
P.O. Box 651
35 Church Street
Lake Placid, NY 12946
Ph: (518) 523-2071
Fax: (518) 523-4106
Website: http://www.usaluge.org
e-mail: staff@usaluge.org

Modern Pentathlon
U.S. Modern Pentathlon Association
530 McCullough
Suite 619
San Antonio, TX 78215
Ph: (210) 246-3000
Fax: (210) 246-3096

Rowing
United States Rowing Association
Pan American Plaza
Suite 400
201 South Capitol Avenue
Indianapolis, IN 46225
Ph: (317) 237-5656
Fax: (317) 237-6546
Website: http://www.coxing.com/usrowing.html
e-mail: usrowing@aol.com

Sailing
United States Sailing Association
P.O. Box 1260
15 Maritime Drive
Portsmouth, RI 02871
Ph: (401) 683-0800
Fax: (401) 683-0840

Shooting
USA Shooting
One Olympic Plaza
Colorado Springs, CO 80909
Ph: (719) 578-4670
Fax: (719) 632-7989
Website: http://www.use.edu/dept/usashooting

Skiing
U.S. Ski and Snowboard Association
P.O. Box 100
1300 Kearns Blvd.
Park City, UT 84060
Ph: (801) 649-9090
Fax: (801) 649-8613
Website: http://www.usskiteam.com

Soccer
U.S. Soccer Federation
U.S. Soccer House
1801-1811 South Prairie Avenue
Chicago, IL 60616
Ph: (312) 808-1300
Fax: (312) 808-1301
Website: http://www.users.aol.com/socfed
e-mail: socfed@aol.com

Softball
Amateur Softball Association
2801 N.E. 50th Street
Oklahoma City, OK 73111
Ph: (403) 424-5266
Fax: (403) 424-3055
Website: http://www.softball.org

Speed Skating
U.S. Speedskating
P.O. Box 16157
Rocky River, OH 44116
Ph: (216) 899-0128
Fax: (216) 899-0109

Swimming
U.S. Swimming, Inc.
One Olympic Plaza
Colorado Springs, CO 80906
Ph: (719) 578-4578
Fax: (719) 578-4669
Website: http://www.usaswim.org

Synchronized Swimming
U.S. Synchronized Swimming, Inc.
Pan American Plaza
Suite 901
201 South Capitol Avenue
Indianapolis, IN 46225
Ph: (317) 237-5700
Fax: (317) 237-5705
Website: www.synchro-usa.org

Table Tennis
USA Table Tennis
One Olympic Plaza
Colorado Springs, CO 80909
Ph: (719) 578-4583
Fax: (719) 632-6071
Website: http://www.usatt.org
e-mail: usatt2@usa.net

Team Handball
U.S. Team Handball Federation
1903 Powers Ferry Road
Suite 230
Atlanta, GA 30339
Ph: (770) 956-7660
Fax: (770) 956-7976
Website: http://www.sport.usa.edu/hansplit.htm
e-mail: usthf@aol.com

Tennis
U.S. Tennis Association
70 West Red Oak Lane
White Plains, NY 10604
Ph: (914) 696-7000
Fax: (914) 696-7167
Website: http://www.usta.com

Track and Field
USA Track & Field
P.O. Box 120
One RCA Dome
Suite 140
Indianapolis, IN 46206
Ph: (317) 261-0500
Fax: (317) 261-0481
Website: http://www.usatf.org

Volleyball
USA Volleyball
3595 East Fountain Blvd.
Suite 1-2
Colorado Springs, CO 80910
Ph: (719) 637-8300
Fax: (719) 597-6307
Website: http://www.volleyball.org/usav

Water Polo
United States Water Polo
1685 West Uintah
Colorado Springs, CO 80904
Ph: (719) 634-0699
Fax: (719) 634-0866
Website: http://www.ewpra.org/uswp
e-mail: uswpoffice@aol.com

Weight Lifting
USA Weightlifting
One Olympic Plaza
Colorado Springs, CO 80909
Ph: (719) 578-4508
Fax: (719) 578-4741
Website: http://www.usaw.org
e-mail: usaw@worldnet.att.net

Wrestling
USA Wrestling
6155 Lehman Drive
Colorado Springs, CO 80918
Ph: (719) 598-8181
Fax: (719) 598-9440
Website: www.usawrestling.org
e-mail: usaw@concentric.net

BIBLIOGRAPHY AND WEBSITES

Bibliography

Alter, Judy. *Stretch and Strengthen*. Boston: Houghton Mifflin, 1986.

American College of Sports Medicine. *Guidelines for Exercise Testing and Prescription*. 5th ed. Baltimore, Md.: Williams and Wilkins, 1995.

American Diabetes Association. *The Fitness Book for People with Diabetes*. Alexandria, Va.: American Diabetes Association, 1994.

American Heart Association. *Fitting in Fitness*. New York: Times Books, 1997.

American Red Cross and U.S. Olympic Committee. *Sport Safety Training Handbook*. St. Louis, Mo.: Mosby Lifeline, 1997.

Anderson, Bob. *Stretching*. Bolinas, Calif.: Shelter Publications, 1997.

————. *Stretching at Your Computer or Desk*. Bolinas, Calif.: Shelter Publications, 1997.

Anderson, Bob, and Bornell, Donald. *Stretch and Strengthen for Rehabilitation and Development*. Palmer Lake, Colo.: Stretching, Inc., 1994.

Anderson, Bob, Burke, Ed, and Pearl, Bill. *Getting in Shape*. Bolinas, Calif.: Shelter Publications, 1998.

Anderson, R. E., Wadden, T. A., Bartlett, S. L., Zemel, B., Verde, Tony J., and Franckowiak, S. C. "Effects of Lifestyle Activity as Structured Aerobic Exercise in Obese Women: A Randomized Trial." *Journal of the American Medical Association* 281, no.4 (1999): 335–340.

Avila, Patrica, and Hovell, Melbourne. "Physical Activity Training for Weight Loss in Latinos: A Controlled Trial." *International Journal of Obesity* 18 (1994): 426–482.

Avila, Vernon L. *Biology: A Human Endeavor*. 1st ed. Jamul, Calif.: Bookmark Publishers, 1992.

Blair, Steven N. *Living with Exercise: Improving Your Health Through Moderate Physical Activity*. Dallas, Tex.: American Health Publishing Co., 1991.

Coleman, E., and Nelson Steen, S. *The Ultimate Sports Nutrition Handbook*. Palo Alto, Calif.: Bull Publishing, 1996.

DeBakey, Michael E., Gotto, A. M., Jr., Scott, L. W., and Foreyt, J. P. *The Living Heart Brand Name Shoppers Guide*. New York: Master Media Limited, 1992.

Dunn, A. L., Marcus, B. H., Kampert, J. B., Garcia, M. E., Kohl, H. W., III, and Blair, S. N. "Comparison of Lifestyle and Structured Intervention to Increase Physical Activity and Cardiorespiratory Fitness: A Randomized Trial." *Journal of the American Medical Association* 281, no. 4 (January 1999): 327–334.

Getchell, Bud, in association with The National Institute for Fitness and Sport. *The Fitness Book*. Carmel, Ind.: Benchmark Press, 1987.

Griffith, H. Winter. *Complete Guide to Sports Injuries*. New York: Putnam-Berkley Group, 1986.

Manson, J., Willett, W., Stampfer, M., Colditz, G., Hunter, D., Hankinson, S., Hennekens, C., and Speizer, F. "Body Weight and Mortality Among Women." *New England Journal of Medicine* 333 (1995): 677–685.

Marieb, Elaine N. *Human Anatomy and Physiology*. 4th ed. Redwood City, Calif.: Benjamin/Cummings Publishing Co., 1998.

Martin, Michael J. *How to Outsmart the Sun: The Ultimate Guide to Healthy, Young-Looking Skin*. San Rafael, Calif.: Penmarin Books, 1993.

Micheli, L. J., and Jenkins, M. *The Sports Medicine Bible*. New York: HarperCollins Publishers, 1995.

Morehouse, Laurence, and Gross, Leonard. *Total Fitness in 30 Minutes a Week*. New York: Pocket Books, 1976.

National Safety Council. *First Aid Handbook*. Boston: Jones and Bartlett Publishers, 1998.

Ornish, Dean. *Program for Reversing Heart Disease*. New York: Ballantine Books, 1990.

Paffenbarger, R. S., Hyde, R. T., Wing A. L., et al. "Physical Activity, All-Cause Mortality, and Longevity of College Alumni." *New England Journal of Medicine* 314 (1986): 605–613.

Pubi, Susan M., Kenney, Patricia M., and Moore, Arch F. *ACSM Fitness Book*. 2d ed. Champaign, Ill.: Human Kinetics, 1998.

Public Health Service, U.S. Department of Health and Human Services. *Clinician's Handbook of Preventive Services: Put Prevention into Family Practice*. Washington, D.C.: Government Printing Office, 1994.

———. *The Surgeon General's Report on Nutrition and Health* (DHHS publication no. DHS 88-50210). Washington, D.C.: Government Printing Office, 1988.

Rippe, J. M., Ward, A., Porcori, H. P., and Freedson, P. S. "Walking for Health and Fitness." *Journal of the American Medical Association* 259 (1988): 2720–2724.

Sharkey, Brian. *Fitness and Health*. 4th ed. Champaign, Ill.: Human Kinetics, 1997.

Shier, David, Butler, Jackie, and Lewis, Ricki. *Hole's Anatomy and Physiology*. 6th ed. Dubuque, Iowa: Wm. C. Brown Publishers, 1996.

Smith, N. J., and Worthington-Roberts, B. *Food for Sport*. Palo Alto, Calif.: Bull Publishing, 1989.

Thibodeau, G. A., and Patton, K. T. *Anthony's Textbook of Anatomy and Physiology*. 15th ed. St. Louis: Mosby-Year Book, 1996.

YMCA. *Y's Way to Physical Fitness: The Complete Guide to Fitness Testing and Instruction*. 3d ed. Champaign, Ill: Human Kinetics, 1989.

Websites

U.S. Olympic Committee
http://www.olympic-usa.org

The Websites for select organizations given below provide information on sports, fitness, and health. These organizations do not diagnose or provide treatment for any disease. Neither the author nor the U.S. Olympic Committee is affiliated with these organizations. Inclusion in this list does not necessarily reflect the views of the author or the USOC, nor does it signify endorsement.

SPORTS AND FITNESS

Fitness Link
http://www.fitnesslink.com

Fitness Online
http://www.fitnessonline.com

Global Health and Fitness
http://www.global-fitness.com

Health and Wellness Resources
http://www.onlinetofitness.com

Index of Sports Medicine and Sports Injuries
http://www.thriveonline.com/health/library/
liu.sports.html

Life Path Health and Wellness
http://www.mylifepath.com

National Association of Governors' Councils
on Physical Fitness and Sports
http://www.fitnesslink.com/Govcouncil

Online Health Fitness and Nutrition
http://ohfn.com

Penmarin Books
http://www.penmarin.com

Shape Up America
http://www2.shapeup.org/sua

Shaping Up the Net
http://www.onlinetofitness.com

HEALTH AND DISEASE PREVENTION

American Cancer Society
http://www.cancer.org

American Dietetic Association
http://www.eatright.org

Arthritis Foundation
http://www.arthritis.org

Centers for Disease Control and Prevention
(CDC)
http://www.cdc.gov

Home Art's Kitchen Counter
http://homearts.com/helpers/calculator/cal-
docfl.htm

National Cancer Institute Cancer Information
Services
http://www.icic.nci.nih.gov

National Health Information Center (NHIC) —
Office of Disease Prevention and Health
Promotion
http://nhic-nt.health.org

National Heart, Lung, and Blood Institute —
Heart Health Information Line
http://www.nih.gov/nhlbi

National Institute on Aging Information Center
http://www.nih.gov/nia

National Mental Health Association
http://www.nmha.com

National Osteoporosis Foundation
http://www.nof.org

ABOUT THE UNITED STATES OLYMPIC COMMITTEE

The United States Olympic Committee (USOC), located in Colorado Springs, Colorado, is a multifaceted organization that serves as the custodian of the United States Olympic movement. More specifically, it is the coordinating body for all Olympic-related activity in the United States.

The mission of the USOC can best be described by the vision and mission statement adopted by the USOC at its February 19, 1997, meeting: "The United States Olympic Committee is dedicated to preparing America's athletes to represent the United States in the ongoing pursuit and achievement of excellence in the Olympic Games and in life. Our Olympians inspire Americans, particularly our youth, to embrace Olympic ideals and to pursue excellence in sports and in their lives."

The mission statement describes the function of the USOC as follows: "The United States Olympic Committee is an organization mandated by Congress under the Amateur Sports Act of 1978 to govern Olympic and Pan American Game–related activities in the USA. The USOC represents athletes, coaches, and administrators of Olympic sport and the American people who support the Olympic movement.

"USOC members include Olympic and Pan American sport organizations

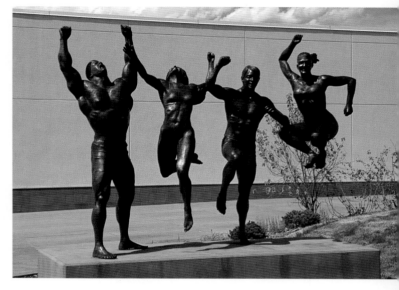

Sculpture of Olympians at the Colorado Springs headquarters of the USOC.

(the national governing bodies), affiliated sport organizations, community-based and education-based multisport organizations, athlete's representatives, armed forces, disabled in sports, state fund-raising organizations, associate members and representatives of the public sector.

"The USOC is governed by a volunteer board of directors and executive committee. The USOC is managed by an executive director with a paid professional staff.

"The USOC is committed to diversity. This means encouraging and recruiting diverse participation in the USOC as an organization as well as in Olympic and Pan American sport."

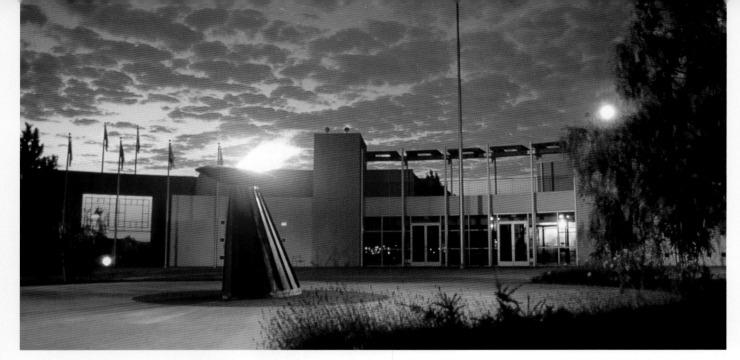

The ARCO Training Center in Chula Vista at night.

Programs

The USOC programs are dedicated to providing quality service and financial support in an integrated program for the benefit of athletes, coaches, and member organizations of the USOC. The U.S. Olympic Committee's programs encompass eight divisions that work together toward the common goal of enhancing athlete development. Despite the shared sense of purpose, each division offers very specialized, distinct services to the National Governing Bodies (NGBs) and other member organizations. The divisions are committed to disseminating information about services through education publications, videos, and seminars.

The eight program divisions are:

➤ Athlete Development Programs

➤ Athlete Support

➤ Coaching

➤ Grants and Planning

➤ National Anti-Doping

➤ Sport Science and Technology

➤ Olympic Training Centers

➤ Sports Medicine

In 1990, the Athlete Development Committee and USOC Board of Directors approved the implementation of pilot Olympic Development Center programs in three cities— Minneapolis/St. Paul, Salt Lake City, and San Antonio. Over the course of the year the USOC will staff this concept and develop programs with youth sports groups in the three cities. At the same time, the USOC will coordinate a broad-based information program on Olympic sports that will allow interested young persons in all areas of the country to find out about Olympic sports and avenues for involvement in their area.

Athlete Support offers three different programs that provide assistance to elite athletes. These programs include athlete grants, employment opportunities, and career and educational assistance.

The Coaching Division is improving both the quality and status of coaching in the U.S. Of particular interest this year are newly designed programs to establish ethical and safety standards for coaches involved with the USOC.

Grants and Planning oversees NGB high-performance planning and the extensive Olympic Grant Program. More than $25 million per year is allocated to support NGB programs.

The primary role of the National Anti-Doping Division is to conduct at-competition and out-of-competition drug testing. The division also promotes education, research, and awareness of drug issues in sport.

The Sports Science and Technology Division seeks to provide national leadership in the application of science to Olympic sport. The program strives to anticipate and meet the sport science and technology needs of Olympic sports in their quest to help elite athletes reach their optimal performance levels.

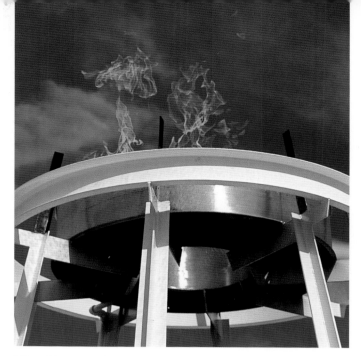

The Olympic flame.

The Olympic Training Centers' staff attempts to provide elite and development athletes with state-of-the-art training facilities. There are four training centers—a training facility in Lake Placid used primarily for winter sports, an all-purpose training center in Colorado Springs, a combined education/training facility at Northern Michigan University, and an all-season training center in Chula Vista, California.

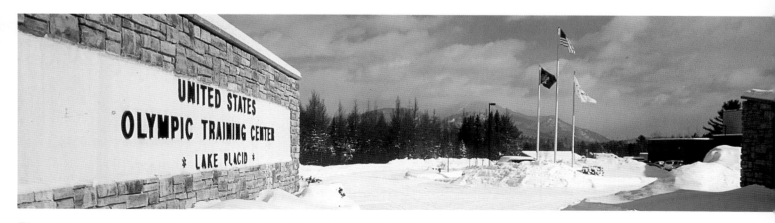

The entry to the U.S. Olympic Training Center at Lake Placid.

THE SPORTS MEDICINE DIVISION

One of the divisions of the USOC is the Sports Medicine Division, located in Colorado Springs and directed by Bob Beeten. The goal of the USOC Sports Medicine Division is to ensure that Olympic athletes and Olympic hopefuls receive the best sports medicine care in a cutting-edge environment, and to serve as a center for the dissemination of information for the Olympic sports community. On a daily basis, the Sports Medicine Division sees and shares the athletes' special moments and the intensity of their emotions in the celebration of victories and the disappointment of losses. Its trainers, physicians, and other health providers are dedicated to providing expert health care necessary to realize the athletes' and America's dreams.

Clinical services program

The Clinical Services Program of the USOC Sports Medicine Division is committed to the promotion of health and excellence in sport. This is accomplished through a comprehensive on-demand health care system for athletes and the provision of research and educational materials. The Clinical Services Program provides health care to athletes at the training centers, as well at the various USOC-supported international games and other competitions.

Medical clinics deliver a combination of acute care, rehabilitation, and physician services. Each Olympic Training Center clinic is furnished with state-of-the-art treatment and rehabilitation equipment. Clinics at international competitions are similarly equipped, emphasizing equipment and supplies for acute care situations.

General medical services include preventive, diagnostic, therapeutic, and short-term rehabilitation to return athletes to activity quickly and safely. The OTC clinics and staff are available to provide elite athletes with comprehensive, long-term rehabilitation programs on an individual basis.

Volunteer program

The USOC medical staff is supplemented by volunteer physicians, chiropractors, and certified athletic trainers. These professionals provide health care services to thousands of athletes at USOC-supported competitions and OTC programs. Selection of the volunteer medical team is a multilevel process that evaluates volunteers on criteria such as medical expertise, interpersonal skills, and adaptability. Volunteers are evaluated by full-time USOC staff during their initial visit to the Olympic Training Centers. Those who perform effectively are invited to serve on the medical staff at additional events. Continued success may eventually lead to

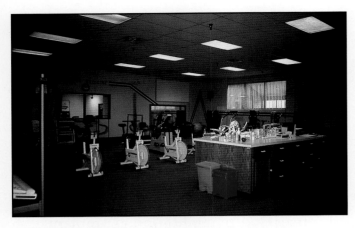

The Sports Medicine Clinic and indoor training facilities at Lake Placid.

participation in international Games. The volunteer medical commitment to the USOC involves a commitment of time ranging from two weeks to eight months or more. This volunteer medical support totals in excess of $13 million each quadrennium.

The USOC Clinical Services Program, in conjunction with the National Athletic Trainers and American Physical Therapy Associations, has established the Elite Sports Medicine and Rehabilitation Network. This service helps elite athletes find athletic trainers and rehabilitation centers close to their training locations. In addition, this network provides athlete trainer resources while teams are training, competing, and traveling around the world. This program will help to reduce health care costs while maintaining optimal medical care for U.S. Olympic–caliber athletes in Olympic and Pan American sports.

Vision care program

A vision care program is offered at the Colorado Springs OTC. Priority is given to Olympic–caliber athletes who are permanent residents of Colorado Springs, and athletes requiring hand-eye or foot-eye coordination for successful sport performance.

Dental services

Recognizing that dental care is integral to health and performance, the USOC Clinical Services Program supports a Dental Services Program aimed at preventing dental problems from interfering with an athlete's training and competition.

Nutrition services

Optimum nutrition is essential to success in sport. However, many athletes give little thought to their eating patterns. The USOC serves as a resource for athletes, coaches, and NGBs by providing nutritional information through educational materials, diet analysis, consultations, lectures, and seminars aimed at the individual needs of different sports. This information can help the athletes optimize their training and performance as well as determine existing or potential nutritional problems.

Common areas of interest include weight loss and gain, precompetition meals, recovery, hydration, and foreign travel. The nutrition program works closely with the USOC food services departments at the Olympic Training Centers to ensure that the best variety of food is available for the athletes. A national network of sports nutrition professionals helps provide support for coaches and athletes in their home training areas throughout the country.

Research

The USOC Clinical Services Program is embarking on research projects in the areas of rehabilitation programs, treatment protocols, and injury statistics. Research will be carried out at the Olympic Training Centers and private facilities. The USOC Sports Medicine Division is launching a pilot project with the National Governing Bodies to enhance its injury surveillance system. Medical personnel traveling with teams will complete injury/illness recording forms. Information from these forms will be compiled by the USOC Sports Medicine Division and returned to NGBs for use in their research and risk management programs.

SportsMed 2000

Being the world leader in program development is both challenging and demanding. However, the United States will continue to be both an innovator and an influential partner within the sports medicine community. Even with state-of-the-art facilities, we must act positively to ensure that we are responsibly affecting healthy athletic performance for athletes at all levels of ability throughout the world and that we continue to improve health care through the prevention and treatment of athletic injuries.

But being a world leader requires far-sighted and uncompromised funding. To this end, the USOC is launching SportsMed 2000, a fund established to further develop USOC leadership and programs of excellence in sports medicine.

SportsMed 2000 goals

- To provide a stable funding source for the Sports Medicine Program
- To create international medical exchanges within the Olympic sports community and Pan American sports organizations
- To better meet and serve the clinical needs of disabled athletes
- To develop a research program on the medical aspects of Olympic, Paralympic, and Pan American sports, using the vast databases available to the USOC
- To collaborate on special education programs that will expand the medical skills which coaches and athletes want from medical staffs
- To enhance both USOC staff and volunteer efforts to deliver the very best sports medicine program available to our athletes

SportsMed 2000 is a plan to establish a working fund of $5 million. Having a stable asset base will enable the USOC to avoid cyclical funding patterns. It will help to ensure a steady flow of funds for proven programs, as well as foster pursuit of experimental or innovative ideas for new programs that will add to the art and science of sports medicine.

The SportsMed 2000 fund will be separately invested and managed by a USOC committee made up of physicians, athletic trainers, business leaders, and investment counselors.

The fund will strive to ensure that the

latest in health care systems, education, research methods, and technology are available and implemented to assist in the success of America's athletes in sports arenas and in life. It will further position the USOC in a role of world leadership in providing health care services for Olympians, Paralympians, and Pan American sports organizations. The fund will ensure the consistent and strategic growth and progress of quality sports medicine into the next century.

INDEX

A

Abdomen, 32
    common injuries, 107–108
    injuries to, 106–107
    strengthening exercises, 64–65
Abductor muscles, 33
Abrasions, 85
Acetaminophen, 76
Achilles tendon, 126, 127
    stretch for, 56
    tear of, 132
Acromioclavicular joint, 94–95
Adductor muscles, 33
Aerobic fitness, 19, 26–27
    benefits of, 28–29
    training guidelines, 31
Aerobic shoes, 158
Age and body fat, average values for, 144
AIDS, 162
Alcoholic beverages, 154
Alternating elbow/knee abdominal curls, 65
Amateur Sports Act of 1978, 173
American College of Sports Medicine, 20
American Physical Therapy Association, 178
Anabolic steroids, 59
Ankles
    anatomy of, 126–127
    common injuries, 128–134
    preventing injuries, 127
    sprains, 133–134
    stretching, 57
Antagonistic muscle groups, 32
Anterior compartment syndrome, 129, 131–132
Anterior cruciate ligament, 119, 120, 122
    rupture of, 135
Archery, 63
Arch stretches, 57
Arms. *See also* Forearms
    combination arm and leg lift, 69
    injuries to, 99–103
    strengthening exercises, 61, 62–63
Arthroscopy of knee, 125
Asthma, 21
Asymmetrical moles, 155–156
Atlas, 99
Alveolar sac, 29
Axis, 99

B

Back. *See also* Lower back; Upper back
    strengthening exercises, 60
Balance, loss of, 73
Baseball finger, 105
Baseball injuries, 98
Basketball
    impingement injuries, 99
    injuries from, 117
Beans in food pyramid, 148
Belly breathing, 159
Biceps
    curls, 62
    strengthening exercises, 62
Biceps brachii muscle, 32
Biceps femoris muscle, 115
Bicycling
    piriformis syndrome, 113
    preventing injuries, 115, 116
    selecting bikes, 118
Bioelectric impedance, 39
Black eyes, 92
Bleeding, 85
Blisters, 84
Blood
    infectious diseases, preventing, 162–163
    water in, 153
Blunt force trauma, 107–108
Body building, 59
Body composition, 19, 38–39
Body fat, average values for, 144
Body Mass Index (BMI), 39, 142–143
Body shaping, 37
Body weight tables, 142–146
Bones, 18. *See also* Fractures; Stress fractures
    dislocations, 83
Borkhuis, Michelle, 60
Brain health, 44
Bray, G. A., 39
Breads
    in food pyramid, 148
    nutrition in, 41
Breakfast sample menus, 149
Breast examinations, 161
Breathing
    belly breathing, 159
    difficulties, 85

techniques, 44, 159
    while stretching, 49
Broken bones. *See* Fractures
Buddies, 21
Bursa, 120
Bursitis, 80

C

Calcaneal tendon. *See* Achilles tendon
Calcaneus, 126, 127
Calcium, 152
Calories, 37
    consumption recommendations, 145–146
    food choices and, 42
Camaraderie, 12–13
Carbohydrates, 43
    endurance and, 36
Cardiac muscle, 78
Carotid pulse, 24
Carpals, 100
Cereals in food pyramid, 148
Cheese in food pyramid, 148
Chest
    muscle strains, 98
    strengthening exercises, 61
    stretches, 51
Chlamydia screening, 161
Cholesterol tests, 161
Chromium, 152
Clinical Services Program (USOC), 179
Clothing
    protective clothing, 115
    workout apparel, 157–158
Comminuted fractures, 82
Common Soft Tissue Injuries chart, 78, 80–81
Compartment syndrome, 129, 131–132
Concussions, 90
Contact sports, 73
Contusions, 80
Convenience of exercise, 27
Cool–down period, 31
Coordination, loss of, 73
Copper, 152
Coracobrachialis muscle, 100–101
Coronary arteries, 26
Coronary collaterals, 26
Cramping, 34, 81
Cranial bones, 88
Cross training, 128

D

Dairy foods in food pyramid, 148
Danielson, Steve, 67

DeBolt, Courtney, 93
Deep breathing, 44
Deltoid muscle, 96, 100–101
Dental services (USOC), 178
Desirable weights for men/women, 144
Diabetes, 38
Diaphragm, 44
Dinner sample menus, 150
Diphtheria immunization, 161
Direct trauma, 73
Dirksen, Emily, 53, 105
Discus throwing, 57
Dislocations, 83
Diving, 2
    back injuries, 112
Drugs, USOC and, 175

E

Eggs in food pyramid, 148
Elbow stretches, 102
Electrolytes, 34
Elite Sports Medicine and Rehabilitation Network, 178
Emotional health, 44–45
Endurance, 19
Energy balance, 37
Erector spinal muscles, 109
Extensor muscles, 33, 89
External abdominal oblique muscles, 106
Eye injuries, 92

F

Fats
    in food pyramid, 148
    metabolizing fat, 25
    nutrition in, 41
Feet
    anatomy of, 126–127
    blisters, 84
    common injuries, 128–134
    preventing injuries, 127
    runner's knee and overpronation, 123
    stretches, 57
Female masculinization, 59
Femur, 113, 119
    fracture of, 118
Fibula, 119
Fibular collateral ligament, 119, 120
    rupture injury, 125
Field hockey, 67
Fingers
    injuries, 105
    strengthening, 62
Fish in food pyramid, 148

Fissured fractures, 82
Fitness assessment, 22–23
FIT program, 16, 31–32
    strengthening exercises, 59
Fitzpatrick, Kevin, 57
Flexibility, 19
    stretching for, 48
Flexor muscles, 33
Fluoride, 152
FOBT (stool sample), 161
Folacin, 151
Food pyramid, 40–41, 147–148
Forearms
    bones of, 101
    strengthening, 62–63
Fractures, 82–83. *See also* Stress fractures
    femur fracture, 118
    of lower leg, 128
    wrist fractures, 104
Free weights, 35
French curl, 62
Frequency of strength training, 59
Fruits
    in food pyramid, 148
    nutrition in, 41
Full push–ups, 61

G

Gamekeeper thumb, 105
Gastrocnemius muscle, 34, 126–127
Gender. *See also* Weight control
    body fat, average values for, 144
    preventive medicine guidelines by, 160
Glenohumeral joint, 94–95
Gluteus maximus muscle, 113
Gluteus medius muscle, 113
Gluteus minimus muscle, 113
Glycogen, 36, 43
Goals, 20–21
    personal fitness plan goals, 135
Golf
    injuries from, 111
    lower back injuries and, 111
Golfer's elbow, 103–104
Gray, D. S., 39
Greenstick fractures, 82
Groin stretches, 55
Gymnastics, 4, 6
    back injuries, 112
    injuries, 106
    piriformis syndrome, 113

H

Half sit–ups, 64
Hamstring muscles, 115
    bicycling and, 115
    strains, 117–118
    strengthening, 115
    stretch, 54
Hands
    bones of, 100
    strengthening, 62
Head
    anatomy of, 88–89
    common injuries, 90–93
    contusions, 90–91
    follow–up guidelines for injuries, 92
    preventing injuries, 89
Hearing exams, 161
Heart
    structure of, 26
Target Heart Rate Zone, 22, 23
Heart disease
    anabolic steroids and, 59
    weight gain and, 38
Heat–related illness, 85, 153
Heat stress, 153–154
    preventing, 154
Heat stroke, 85, 153
Heel spurs, 133
Height measurements, 161
Helmets, 89
    for in–line skaters, 92–93
Hematoma, 80
    of thigh, 116
Hepatitis, preventing, 161
Heptathlon, 21
Heredity, 25
Hernias, 108
High blood pressure, 18
    anabolic steroids and, 59
    weight and, 38, 161
Hips
    common injuries, 110–113
    injuries to, 109–113
    leg lifts for, 67
    preventing injuries, 110
    strengthening exercises, 66–67
    stretches, 53, 55
HIV infection, preventing, 162
Human skeleton, 74
Hurdles, 23
Hydration, 153–154

I

Ibuprofen, 76
Iliac crest of pelvis, 113
Illiocostalis cervicis muscle, 109
Illiocostalis lumborum muscle, 109
Illiocostalis thoracis muscle, 109
Impact and exercise, 27
Impingement syndrome, 98–99
Improvements, monitoring, 25
Inflammation, 80
Influenza immunization, 161
Infraspinatus muscle, 95–96
Inguinal ligament, 106
Injuries, 72–74. *See also* Rehabilitation
    abrasions, 85
    blisters, 84
    caring for, 76
    defined, 73–74
    heat–related illness, 85
    hip injuries, 109–113
    insect bites, 85
    internal bleeding, 85
    lacerations, 84
    lower back injuries, 109–113
    prevention of, 77
    severity ratings, 74–75
    sunburn, 84–85
In–line skating, 92–93
Insect bites, 85
Intensity of exercise, 59
Internal bleeding, 85
International Olympic Committee, 59. *See also* United
    States Olympic Committee
Iodine, 152
Iron, 152
Isokinetic exercises, 58
Isometric exercises, 58
Isotonic exercises, 58

J

Jogging. *See* Running
Joints
    problems, 18
    subluxation, 83
Joyner–Kersee, Jackie, 21
Jumper's knee, 123–124
Jumping, 129

K

Kelly, Pete, 65
Knee
    anatomy of, 119
    common injuries, 122–125

    injuries to, 119–125
    preventing injuries, 120–122
    push–ups, 61

L

Lacerations, 84
Lactic acid, 34
Lateral collateral ligament, 119, 120
    rupture injury, 125
Lateral condyle, 119
Lateral epicondylitis, 73, 102
Lateral meniscus, 119
    torn lateral meniscus, 125
Latissimus dorsi muscle, 96, 100–101, 109
Legs
    anatomy of, 126–127
    combination arm and leg lift, 69
    common injuries, 128–134
    leg raises, 68
    lower leg stretches, 56–57
    preventing injuries, 127
    shin pain, 128–129
    strengthening exercises, 66–67
    stress fractures, 129, 130
    toe lifts, 68
    upper leg stretches, 54–55
Ligament of Wrisberg, 119
Ligaments, 74
    strains, 81
    Wrisberg, ligament of, 119
Liver, anabolic steroids and, 59
Longissimus capitis muscle, 109
Longissimus cervicis muscle, 109
Longissimus thoracis muscle, 109
Lower back
    common injuries, 110–113
    injuries to, 109–113
    preventing injuries, 110
    strains, 110–111
    stretches for, 52–53
Lumbar pain, 113
Lunch sample menus, 149
Lung capacity, 28–29
Lying hip raise, 66
Lymph, 153

M

Magnesium, 152
Malahy, Jo–Ann, 63
Male reproductive diseases, 59
Mallet finger, 105
Mammograms, 161
Manganese, 152
Massage, 34

Maturity, 25
Measles immunization, 161
Meats
    in food pyramid, 148
    nutrition in, 41
Medial collateral ligament, 120
Medial condyle, 119
Medial epicondylitis, 103–104
Medial meniscus, 119
Medial tibial pain syndrome, 129–130
Melanoma, 155–156
Menisci, 119
Mental health, 44–45
Metropolitan Life Weight Tables, 39, 144–146
    body fat, average values for, 144
    Calorie consumption recommendations, 145–146
    desirable weights for men/women, 144
Milk
    in food pyramid, 148
    nutrition in, 41
Minerals, RDA for, 152
MMR immunization, 161
Moderately intense activity, 20
Moe, Tommy, 134
Moles, checking on, 155–156
Mosley, Benita Fitzgerald, 23
Motivation hurdle, 21
Muhammad, Sabir, 99
Mumps immunization, 161
Muscles
    abdominal muscles, 106–107
    contraction, 34
    cramping, 34, 81
    neck muscles, 89
    soft tissue injuries, 74
    strains, 81
    types of, 78
Muscular strength/endurance, 19, 36
Muscular system, 33

N

National Athletic Trainers, 178
National Governing Bodies (NGBs), 174
Neck
    anatomy of, 88–89
    common injuries, 90–93
    pain in, 92–93
    preventing injuries, 89
    stretches, 50, 89
Niacin, 151
Nose bleeds, 91–92
Nutrition, 25
    endurance and, 36
    food choices, 42–43

food pyramid, 40–41, 147–148
    sample menus, 149–150
    USOC services, 178–179
    weight control and, 147–152
Nuts in food pyramid, 148

O

Oblique fractures, 82
Oerter, Al, 108
Oils
    in food pyramid, 148
    nutrition in, 41
Olympic Development Center, 174–175
Olympic Training Centers, 175
100–meter hurdles, 23
Overall body stretch, 49
Overhead extensions, 62
Overpronation of foot, 123
Over–the–counter medication, 76
Oxygen, 26
    muscle contraction and, 34
    respiratory system and, 28–29
    transportation of, 28

P

Pain. See Injuries
Pan American sports organizations, 173
Pap smears, 161
Paralympics, 179–180
Pasta in food pyramid, 148
Patella, 34, 114, 119, 120
Patellar ligament, 120
Patellar tendinitis (jumper's knee), 123–124
Patellar tendon, 114
Patello–femoral pain (runner's knee), 123
Pear shape, 38
Pectoralis major muscle, 96, 100–101
Pelvic girdle, 109
Pelvis, 109
    iliac crest of, 113
Performance goals, 20
Peroneus longus muscle, 34
Personal fitness plan, 135–141
    body shaping log, 141
    examples of, 137–138
    muscular fitness log, 140
    stretching log, 139
Phalanges, 127
Phosphorus, 152
Piriformis muscle, 113
Piriformis syndrome, 113
Plantar arch, 127
Plantar fascia, 127

Plantar fasciitis, 132–133
Pneumococcal immunization, 161
Posterior cruciate ligament, 119, 120, 122
Posterior oblique ligament, 120
Posture, 112
Potassium, 152
Pot bellies, 38
Poultry in food pyramid, 148
President's Council on Physical Fitness, 20
Prevention of injuries, 77
Preventive medicine guidelines, 160–161
Prostate, 59
Protective pads, 115
Protein, 43
Pulmonary arterioles, 29
Pulmonary venules, 29
Pulse rate, 24–25
Push–ups, 61
Pyridoxine, 151

Q

Quadratus femoris muscle, 113
Quadriceps muscles, 114–115
    bicycling and, 115
    chair leg raises, 66
    patella and, 120
    stretching of, 55, 115

R

Race walking, 54
Racket sports, 99
Radial pulse, 24
Radius, 100, 101
Recommended daily allowance (RDA), 151–152
Rectal exams, 161
Rectus abdominis muscle, 106
Rectus femoris muscle, 114
Rehabilitation
    goal of, 86
    of lower leg, 127
Relaxation, 45
    techniques, 159
Repetitive motion injuries, 72–73
Research program (USOC), 179
Resources, list of, 163–165
Respiratory system, 28–29
Rest
    muscle soreness, 34
    muscular fatigue and, 34
    need for, 25
Reverse fly, 60
Reverse wrist curl, 102
Rhomboideus major muscle, 109

Rice in food pyramid, 148
RICE (Rest, Ice, Compression, and Elevation), 76, 87
    shoulder injuries, 96
Rotator cuff muscles, 96
    impingement syndrome, 98–99
    injury to, 97–98
Rotator cuff tendinitis, 62
Rowing, 53, 60
Rubber ball squeeze, 62
Rubella immunization, 161
Runner's knee, 73, 123
Running, 8
    knee injuries, 73, 120, 123
    medial tibial pain syndrome, 129
    preventing injuries, 130–131
    stress fractures, 83
Running shoes, 158
Ruptured knee ligaments, 125

S

Saliva, 153
Sartorius muscle, 114–115
Scalp wounds, 90
Scapulothoracic joint, 94–95
Sciatica, 112–113
Scott, Tyrone, 113
Scovel, Sally, 51
Seaman, Tim, 54
Selenium, 152
Semimembranosus muscle, 115
Semispinalis capitis muscle, 89, 109
Semispinalis thoracis muscle, 109
Semitendinosus muscle, 115
Severity of injuries, 75
Shin guards, 127
Shin pain, 128–129
Shin splints, 73, 128
Shoes, 31, 157–158
    preventing injuries and, 127
    walking shoes, 77
Shoulders
    anatomy of, 94–96
    common injuries, 97–99
    exercises for, 36
    preventing injuries, 96–97
    strengthening exercises, 60
    stretches, 50, 51
Sigmoidoscopy, 161
Silence, 45
Sitting calf stretch, 56
Sit–ups, 64
Skeletal injuries, 73, 74, 82–84
Skeletal muscles, 79
Skeleton, 74

Skiing, 27
    anterior cruciate ligament injuries, 125
    injuries from, 123
    knee injuries and, 124
    lower leg injuries, 127
    protective clothing, 115
Skill factors, 27
Skinfold measurement, 39
Ski pole thumb, 105
Skull, 88
Sleeping, 25, 110
Smooth muscle, 78–79
Snacks, sample menus, 149
Snowboarding, 10
    injuries, 104
    injuries from, 123
Snow skiing. *See* Skiing
Soccer
    injuries from, 121
    shin guards for, 127
Social factors, 27
Softball injuries, 98
Soft tissue injuries, 73–74, 78–81
Soleus muscle, 126, 127
Soreness, 34
Specialty shoes, 158
SPF factors, 155
Spinalis thoracis muscle, 109
Spine, 109
Spiral fractures, 82
Splenius capitis muscle, 89, 109
Splenius cervicis muscle, 109
Spondylosis, 112–113
Spondylolisthesis, 112–113
Spongy disks, 109
SportsMed 2000 (USOC), 179–180
Sports Medicine Division (USOC)
    Clinical Services Program, 177
    dental services, 178
    nutrition services, 178–179
    research program, 180
SportsMed 2000, 179–180
    vision care program, 178
    volunteer program, 177–178
Sprains
    ankle sprains, 133–134
    healing time for, 82
Standing calf stretch, 56
Sternoclavicular joint, 94–95
Sternocleidomastoid muscle, 89
Steroids, anabolic, 59
Stool sample (FOBT), 161
Strains
    hamstring strains, 117–118
    thigh strains, 116

Street, Picabo, 124
Strengthening exercises, 8–9, 19, 58–69
    abdominals, 64–65
    arms, 61, 62–63
    back and shoulders, 60
    chest, 61
    combination exercises, 69
    hips, 66–67
    legs, 66–67
    program for, 59
Strength training
    guidelines, 35
    muscular fitness and, 32
Stress and injury, 72
Stress fractures, 83–84
    of lower leg, 129, 130
Stretching, 31
    for flexibility, 48
    legs, 54–57
    overall body stretch, 49
    of quadriceps, 115
    swimming and, 95
    technique for, 49
    upper body stretches, 50–51
Subluxation, 83
Subscapularis muscle, 95–96
Summer workout clothes, 157
Sunburn, 84–85
    preventing, 155–156
Sunscreens, 85, 155
Supraspinatus muscle, 95–96
Sweating, 153
Sweets
    in food pyramid, 148
    nutrition in, 41
Swimming, 27
    impingement injuries, 99
    preventing injuries, 95

T

Target Heart Rate Zone, 22, 23
    exercising within, 24–25
Teamwork, 12–13
Tendinitis, 80
    of Achilles tendon, 132
    shoulder tendinitis, 97
Tendon strain, 81
Tennis
    injuries, 102–103
    rackets, selecting, 103
Tennis elbow, 73, 102
Teres major muscle, 100–101
Teres minor muscle, 95–96
Testicles, 59

Tetanus immunization, 161
Thiamin, 151
Thigh
    anatomy of, 114
    injuries to, 114–118
    preventing injuries, 115–116
    strains, 116
Thigh common injuries, 116–118
Thighs
    leg raises, 68
Thumb injuries, 105
Tibia, 126
Tibial collateral ligament, 119
Tibialis anterior muscle, 34, 126
Tibial tuberosity, 119
Tibula, 119
Time hurdles, 21
Toe lifts, 68
Torn knee ligaments, 125
Transverse fractures, 82
Transverse ligament of knee, 119, 120
Trapezius muscle, 96
Triceps muscle, 32
    strengthening exercises, 62
    stretches, 51
Tuberculin tests, 161

U

Ulna, 100, 101
Underwater body weighing, 39
United States Olympic Committee, 173–176. *See also*
        Sports Medicine Division (USOC)
Athlete Development Committee, 174
Athlete Support, 174–175
Coaching Division, 175
Grants and Planning, 175
National Anti–Doping Division, 175
    programs of, 174–175
Upper back
    strains, 98
    stretches for, 50–51, 51
Upper extremities, injuries to, 99–103
Urine, color of, 153

V

Vastus intermedius muscle, 114
Vastus lateralis muscle, 114
Vastus medialis muscle, 114
Vegetables in food pyramid, 148
Ventilation, 28
Vertebrae, 99

spongy disks, 109
Vision care (USOC), 178
Vision exams, 161
Visualization techniques, 159
Vitamin A, 151
Vitamin B_1, 151
Vitamin B_6, 151
Vitamin B_{12}, 151
Vitamin C, 151
Vitamin D, 151
Vitamin E, 151
Vitamin K, 151
Vitamins, RDA for, 151
Volunteer program (USOC), 177–178

W

Waist–to–hip ratio (WHR), 38–39
Walking
    knee injuries, 120
    preventing injuries, 130–131
    program, 31
Walking shoes, 77, 158
Warm–ups, 88
Water, 25
    endurance and, 36
    in FIT program, 31
    heat stress and, 153–154
Weight control, 37
    body fat, average values for, 144
    Calorie consumption recommendations, 145–146
    desirable weights for men/women, 144
    in FIT program, 31
    nutrition and, 147–152
    tables for body weight, 142–146
Weight lifting, 99
Weight machines, 35
Weights, 59
Wheelchair racing, 7
Wilson, Blaine, 118
Winter workout clothes, 157
Wrist
    bones, 100
    fractures, 104–105
    strains/sprains, 103
    strengthening, 62
    strengthening exercises, 101–102
Wrist curl, 101

Z

Zinc, 152

CREDITS

Illustrations

Pages 24, 26, 31, 34, 37, 38, 39, 40, 42, 74 top, 77, 82, 83, 95, 96, 102, 104, 109, 113, 119 right, 120, 122, 123, 125, 127, 131, 132, and 133 by Elizabeth Morales.

Pages 28, 32, 33, and 44 from Vernon L. Avila, *Biology: A Human Endeavor*, Bookmark Publishers (Chula Vista, Ca., 1992). Reprinted by permission.

Pages 74 bottom, 94, 100, and 114 from *Human Anatomy & Physiology*, by Elaine Marieb; © 1989, Benjamin/Cummings Publishing Company, Inc. Reprinted by permission.

Pages 78, 79, 88, 97, 101, 106, 119 bottom, and 126 from Gary Thibodeau and Kevin Patton, *Anthony's Textbook of Anatomy and Physiology, 15th edition*, Mosby-Year Book, Inc. (St. Louis, Mo., 1996). Reprinted by permission.

Photographs

PART I   Page 1: Digital Stock. Pages 2–3: 1992 Allsport USA/Bob Martin. Pages 4–5: Digital Stock. Page 6: 1996 Allsport USA/D. Reinzinger. Page 7: Digital Stock. Page 9: 1996 Allsport USA/Mike Hewitt. Pages 10–11: © 1999, Comstock, Inc. Pages 12–13: © 1999, Comstock, Inc. Page 14: 1998 Allsport USA/Al Bello. Page 15: 1998 Allsport USA/Al Bello.

PART II   Page 16: Scott Gardner. Page 18: © 1999, Comstock, Inc. Page 19: Tony Stone Images. Page 20 both: © 1999, Comstock, Inc. Page 21 top: 1993, Allsport USA/Tony Duffy. Page 21 bottom: Scott Gardner. Page 23: courtesy of Benita Fitzgerald. Page 24: Al Bruton. Page 25: © 1999, Comstock, Inc. Page 26: Al Bruton. Page 27 all: © 1999, Comstock, Inc. Page 29 top: Bill Longcore/Photo Researchers, Inc. Page 29 bottom: Al Bruton. Page 31: © 1999, Comstock, Inc. Page 30 both: © 1999, Comstock, Inc. Page 33: courtesy of Bob Beeten, USOC. Page 34: courtesy of Bob Beeten, USOC. Page 36 top left and bottom: Al Bruton. Page 36 right: courtesy of Bob Beeten, USOC. Page 39: © 1999, Comstock, Inc. Page 41 all: © 1999, Comstock, Inc. Page 43 top: Al Bruton. Page 43 bottom: © 1999, Comstock, Inc. Page 45: © 1999, Comstock, Inc.

PART III   Pages 46–47: 1998 Allsport USA/Kellie Landis. Page 48: © 1999, Comstock, Inc. Page 49 top: Image Bank. Page 49 bottom: David Knoll. Page 50 right: Al Bruton. Page 50 left: David Knoll. Page 51 box: courtesy of Sally Scovel. Page 51: Vernon Avila. Page 52: Al Bruton. Page 53 box: courtesy of Karen Dunne. Page 53: David Knoll. Page 54 box: courtesy of Tim Seaman. Pages 54–55: David Knoll. Page 56: Vernon Avila. Page 57 box: courtesy of Kevin Fitzpatrick. Page 57: Al Bruton. Page 58: © 1999, Comstock, Inc. Page 59: © 1999, Comstock, Inc. Page 60 box: courtesy of Michelle Borkhuis. Page 60: Al Bruton. Page 61: David Knoll. Page 62 top: Al Bruton. Page 62 bottom: David Knoll. Page 63 box: courtesy of Jo-Ann Malahy. Pages 63–65: Al Bruton. Page 65 box: 1999 Allsport USA/Simon Bruty. Page 66 top: Al Bruton. Page 66 bottom and page 67 top: David Knoll. Page 67 box: courtesy of Steve Danielson. Page 68 top: David Knoll. Page 68 bottom and page 69: Al Bruton.

PART IV   Pages 70–71: © TSM/ Michael Daly. Page 72: 1997 Allsport USA/Clive Brunskill. Page 73 left: Jim Cummins/FPG International LLC. Page 73 right: 1998 Allsport USA/Glace Hommes. Page 76: Mark Adams/FPG International LLC. Page 77 left: Jim Cummins/FPG International LLC. Page 77 right: David Knoll. Page 83: John Terence Turner/FPG International LLC. Page 84 top: © 1999, Comstock, Inc. Page 84 bottom: © TSM/David Stoecklin. Page 86: Jim Cummins/FPG International LLC. Page 87 top: © 1999,Comstock, Inc. Page 87 bottom: Jim Cummins/FPG International LLC. Page 89: Scott Markewitz/FPG International LLC. Page 90: 1996 Allsport USA/John Todd. Page 91 top: © 1999, Comstock, Inc. Page 91 bottom: 1988 Allsport USA/R. Cheyne. Page 93: courtesy of Courtney DeBolt. Page 98: Scott Gardner. Page 99 left: Scott Gardner. Page 99 box: 1998 Allsport USA/Todd Warshaw. Pages 101–103: David Knoll. Page 104: VCG/FPG International LLC. Page 105: © Joel W. Rogers, Seattle. Page 106: Ed Braveman/FPG International LLC. Page 107: 1998 Allsport USA/Brian Bahr. Page 108 top: 1996 Allsport USA/Doug Pensinger. Page 108 box: © Allsport. Page 110: Al Bruton. Page 111 left: Ron Chapple/FPG International, LLC. Page 111 right: Jim Cummins/FPG International, LLC. Page 112 left: 1996 Allsport USA/Simon Bruty. Page 112 right: 1996 Allsport USA/J. Vaugust. Page 113 box: courtesy of Tyrone Scott. Page 115: Jim Cummins/FPG International LLC. Page 116 top: Scott Gardner. Page 116 bottom: Al Bruton. Page 117: Scott Gardner. Page 118 box: 1996 Allsport USA/Mike Powell. Page 121: 1996 Allsport USA/Clive Brunskill. Page 122: Jim Cummins/FPG International LLC. Page 124 top right: 1995 Allsport USA/Otto Gruele. Page 124 box: 1996 Allsport USA/Mike Powell. Page 124 bottom: Scott Gardner. Page 125: courtesy of Heinz Hoenecke, Jr., M.D. Page 127: © 1999, Comstock, Inc. Page 128: © Jon Feingersh/TSM. Page 129: 1996 Allsport USA/Stu Forster. Page 132: David Knoll. Page 133: 1992 Allsport USA/James Meehan. Page 130: Jim Cummins/FPG International LLC. Page 134: 1997 Allsport USA/Simon Bruty.

Appendixes Pages 155–156: courtesy of The Skin Cancer Foundation, New York, NY, ©1985. Page 173: Scott Gardner. Page 175: © Allen Kennedy. Pages175 bottom and 178: courtesy of the U.S. Olympic Committee.